PENGUIN BOOKS

CRAZYWATER

Brian Maracle is an award-winning journalist and a member of the Mohawk Nation, originally from the Six Nations Grand River Territory near Brantford, Ontario. During the 1970s he worked for native organizations at the local, provincial and national levels, and since the early 1980s he has worked as a print and broadcast journalist, specializing in native issues. He is a former host of the CBC Radio program, *Our Native Land*, and a former reporter for *The Globe and Mail*. He recently returned to live on the Six Nations Grand River Territory.

CRAZYWATER

Native Voices on Addiction and Recovery

BRIAN MARACLE

Penguin Books

PENGUIN BOOKS
Published by the Penguin Group
Penguin Books Canada Ltd, 10 Alcorn Avenue, Toronto, Ontario, Canada M4V 3B2
Penguin Books Ltd, 27 Wrights Lane, London W8 5TZ, England
Penguin Books USA Inc., 375 Hudson Street, New York, New York 10014, U.S.A.
Penguin Books Australia Ltd, Ringwood, Victoria, Australia
Penguin Books (NZ) Ltd, 182-190 Wairau Road, Auckland 10, New Zealand

Penguin Books Ltd, Registered Offices:
Harmondsworth, Middlesex, England

First published in Viking by Penguin Books Canada Limited, 1993

Published in Penguin Books, 1994

10 9 8 7 6 5 4 3 2 1

Copyright © Brian Maracle, 1993

Manufactured in Canada

Canadian Cataloguing in Publication Data
Maracle, Brian, 1947–
    Crazywater

ISBN 0-14-017287-4

1. Indians of North America - Alcohol use. 2. Native peoples - Canada - Alcohol use.
3. Alcoholics - Rehabilitation. I. Title.

E98.L7M37 1994   362.29'2'08997   C92-095777-3

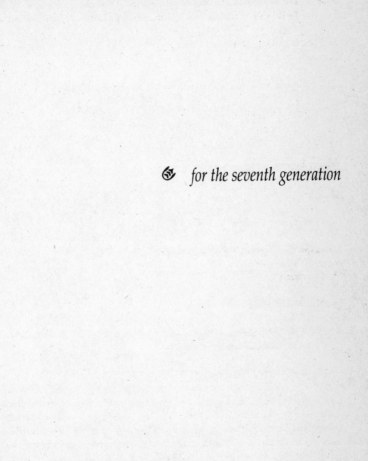 *for the seventh generation*

ACKNOWLEDGMENTS

Many of the people I interviewed for this book asked to have their names withheld and their identity protected, so I have changed names, locations and other identifying characteristics. In some cases, I have used a speaker's native name at their request. While some speakers said they would be proud to have their full name published, others wanted only their first name used, in accordance with the first-name-only practice of Alcoholics Anonymous. In a few cases, I have changed names of different speakers who had the same name, to eliminate confusion.

In any case, the names and identities of the speakers in this book are not important. Their stories are. I have identified all the speakers in *Crazywater* by just one name to focus attention, not on a few individuals, but on stories and experiences shared by all native people. The age of each speaker mentioned in *Crazywater*, incidently, is accurate as of the date of the interview.

The spellings of various native language words were often provided by the speaker and are not meant to be definitive, since the spellings (and the words themselves) vary from place to place and speaker to speaker.

My idea for the book is rooted in the fact that native wit and wisdom is largely unknown and unappreciated — so I have used the oral history format to let the people tell their own stories and bring their talents to light. Interviews have been edited to retain as much of the speaker's grammar, vocabulary, accent and pacing as possible. I can't think of a better way to get the reader to share our shame, pain, anger, joy and celebration.

I could not have completed this work without the help I received from hundreds of people and agencies. The list includes dozens of native friendship centres, native radio stations and native organizations which advertised my project. As well, the directors and staff at Stoney Medicine Lodge, St. Paul's Treatment Centre, Poundmaker's Lodge and Nelson House Medicine Lodge helped me in ways too numerous to mention.

I received valuable information, introductions, suggestions, translations and feedback from: Solomon Awashish, Basil Johnston, Carman Maracle, Rhonda McBride, Daniel David Moses, Cindy Peltier, Dave Thompson and Geoffrey York. From the very outset, Jackie Kaiser at Penguin Books Canada was unfailingly enthusiastic and helpful in providing encouragement and much-needed editorial guidance.

Financial assistance for this project was provided by the National Native Alcohol and Drug Abuse Program of Health and Welfare Canada and by the Explorations Program of the Canada Council. Diane Kaplan and the Alaska Public Radio Network provided me with travel assistance as did Ken Williams and the Native Friendship Centre of Montreal.

The greatest contribution of all, however, came from the hundreds of native people who shared their time, stories and emotions so graciously and generously. Lastly, I want to acknowledge the love and support of my wife Dora, our daughter Zoe, and my parents and family on both shores of Great Turtle Island.

To everyone who helped me in so many ways, I owe a "very big thank you" — *Niawenkowa*.

Brian Maracle
Ottawa, Ontario
July 1992

TERMINOLOGY

aboriginal A term that should be used only as an adjective to describe individuals or mixed groups of Indian, Metis or Inuit people. Wrongly used by the news media as a noun, as in: "The aboriginals are . . ." The proper usage is: "The aboriginal *people* (or *peoples*) are . . ." (See *native*.)

Anishinaubaequae The term that Ojibway-speaking peoples use to describe their women; literally, "a good being [female]."

Blackfeet / Blackfoot The members of this Indian nation who live north of the forty-ninth parallel prefer to be called Blackfoot. Their cousins south of the border prefer to be called Blackfeet.

Dene The Indian peoples of the Northwest Territories, parts of the Yukon and the northern portions of the prairie provinces; literally, "the people." They include the Chipewyan, Dogrib, Slavey and Gwich'in peoples.

drag, the The downtown / skid-row section of western Canadian cities.

Great Turtle Island North America; the term comes from the Haudenosaunee belief that the world they knew in pre-Columbian times rested on the back of a giant snapping turtle.

Haudenosaunee "The people of the longhouse;" the Iroquois; the people of the six nations of the Iroquois Confederacy – the Mohawk, Oneida, Onondaga, Cayuga, Seneca and Tuscarora.

Indian Despite its conceded unpopularity in many quarters, I use this term in a broad sense to describe people of native Indian ancestry. I only use it in its narrow, legal sense of people with government-recognized Indian "status" when dealing with prohibition under the Indian Act. I never use it to describe non-Indian people who acquired Indian "status" through marriage.

Inuit The term the aboriginal people of the Arctic prefer to be called; literally, "the people."

inuk An Inuit man or woman.

MDA Methylenedioxyamphetamine, a hallucinogen.

medaewaewin An Ojibway term for a person who communicates with the manitous (the spirits) by drumming to obtain their goodwill to heal the sick; literally, "the sound."

Metis Originally, the children and descendants of inter-marriage between Indians and "French-Canadians." Now, a person of mixed Indian-and-white ancestry who identifies him or herself as a Metis.

native A term that should be used only as an adjective, to describe individuals or mixed groups of Indian, Metis or Inuit people. Wrongly used by the media as a noun, as in: "John Smith, a native, said . . ." The proper usage is: "John Smith, a native *man*, said . . ." (See *aboriginal*.)

Onkwehonwe   The term the Haudenosaunee use to describe Indian people or native people in general; literally, "the real people."

Poundmaker's   A well-known native treatment centre on the outskirts of Edmonton. Poundmaker's Lodge is named after a Cree chief who was wrongly imprisoned for taking part in the Riel Rebellion.

sweat lodge   A domed tent-like structure. Heated stones are placed inside the sweat lodge and water is poured on them to produce steam as part of a spiritual or cultural purification ceremony.

sweetgrass   A sweet-smelling grass burned in purification ceremonies; people "wash" themselves in its smoke.

CONTENTS

Introduction 1

1 The Old Days 17

2 Prohibition 44

3 The First Time 58

4 Bingeing, Bootlegging and Racism 74

5 Escape and Aftermath 86

6 Craziness 101

7 Drugs 129

8 Images 140

9 Quitting 149

10 Treatment 176

11 Alcoholics Anonymous 199

12 Reasons 215

13 Solutions 232

14 Sobriety 254

Epilogue 283

CRAZYWATER

INTRODUCTION

"Drink no firewater of the white man. It makes you mice for the white men who are cats. Many a meal they have eaten of you."

— Skenando, Oneida chief, c. 1800

The stories of the seventy-five different people which appear in this book are based on two hundred interviews I did over a three-year period with Onkwehonwe from all parts of Great Turtle Island. I interviewed anyone and everyone — men and women; young people and old people; drinkers and non-drinkers; Indians, Metis and Inuit; reserve residents and city-dwellers; native professionals and welfare recipients.

I asked them to tell me about the first time they drank. I asked them to tell me how they drank and what they liked about it. I asked them about prohibition, bootleggers, homebrew, hangovers, drugs, sobering up, Alcoholics Anonymous, spirituality and sobriety. In short, I asked them to tell me anything and everything about native people and alcohol.

1

hen, is a collection of their stories about our peo-
volvement with alcohol. I interviewed native
peop only because this book is meant to be *our* story. The
non-native academics, social scientists, government
experts and medical authorities have all had their say.
Now it's our turn.

For the past twenty years my work has centred on the
Onkwehonwe. I spent most of the 1970s working for
native organizations at the local, provincial and national
levels, in the fields of education, political development
and communications. In 1981, I began working in the
mainstream media as a reporter for *The Globe and Mail*. The
next year I became the host of the long-running (but now-
dead) CBC Radio program *Our Native Land*. With a shove
from CBC in 1985, I began my career as a freelance writer
and broadcaster, specializing in coverage of native issues.

My work over the past twenty years has allowed me to
see and understand the real problems facing the
Onkwehonwe. Before going any further, let me stress that
alcohol or alcoholism is *not* the problem. Neither is it *the*
greatest problem facing native people today. Alcoholism
is just a symptom of the fundamental problems facing
native people — problems that cannot be solved by half-
measures in isolation. The ultimate resolution of native
alcoholism will require a combination of spiritual, cultural, social, economic and political action. In a sense, it
means that we, as native people, have to become reborn.
We have to become whole once again. And we will have
to deal with our alcoholism before we can deal with other
issues successfully. For example, although our alcoholism
is partly rooted in our powerlessness, self-government

alone will not solve "the problem." What's more, self-government will not live up to its potential, it will not "work," until we are sober, healthy and happy.

The story of my own involvement and my family's involvement with alcohol is similar to many of the stories in this book. My parents and most of my brothers and sisters are now sober, non-drinking people. Ten years ago, though, most of us were boozers and problem drinkers. I myself quit drinking in 1985, and to use a borrowed sports analogy, I still have a high lifetime average.

I began feeling the effects of alcohol from the day I was born because my parents were "non-status" Indians, native people without government-recognized Indian rights. I was not a "status" Indian because my father's father signed away his Indian rights in the early 1920s. At that time it was against the law for Indians to buy or possess alcohol and that was one of the reasons my grandfather relinquished his Indian status — so he could drink. As a result of that decision, my father was never registered as an Indian and when he married my mother, she was stripped of her Indian status. Their seven children then grew up with no Indian rights. (The lack of these rights and government "benefits" was a blessing in some ways, but that's another story.) What it all amounted to, though, was that a total of nine people paid the price over a period lasting more than sixty-five years — all because of one man's love of beer.

My family has felt the effects of alcohol in other ways as well. When I was a boy, one of my cousins stabbed and killed another of my cousins in a drunken argument over a bottle of wine. Another of my cousins was murdered while he was drunk. When I was a teenager, I watched my favourite uncle wither and waste away as he drank himself to death. He died of cirrhosis when he was just thirty-three. When I was older, another of my uncles also died from drinking. He was thirty-seven. One of my aunts died from a lifetime of hard drinking when she was sixty. One of my cousins went to prison for murder after he woke up from a drunk to find a woman dead in his room. My brother-in-law choked to death on his own vomit after he got drunk and passed out. My sister's boyfriend was stabbed to death in a bar-room argument over a chair. (By the way, I haven't mentioned the other effects alcohol has had on my family — the broken marriages, apprehended children, car accidents, fights, broken bones, cuts, scars, arrests and jail terms.)

But when I look back on the death, pain and heartache in my family history and compare it with what other native people have gone through, I consider myself lucky because I know it could have been much, much worse.

So let me also stress here that I have not put *Crazywater* together to rant and rave against the evils of drink, in spite of the effect that drinking has had on me and my family. I am not on a messianic crusade to get native people to quit drinking. I am concerned about native alcoholism in the same way that I am concerned about all the other issues facing native people — racism, land claims, economic development and self-government, to name just a few. I am concerned about each and every one of these issues but I am not maniacally obsessed with any one of them.

If *Crazywater* is anything, then, it is this: It is just part of my overall effort — which in turn is part of many people's overall efforts — to rejuvenate our people, to make ourselves whole once again, to heal our pain, to create social justice and strengthen our language, culture and traditions. *Crazywater* tells about one of the major problems our people face, the recovery our people have made and the healing we must still undergo.

🐚

If there is one image about native people and alcohol that most Canadians have in their minds, it probably involves an incident that goes something like this:

You are walking on a downtown street in a major Canadian city. You are one of dozens of shoppers and office workers filling the sidewalk. Everyone is striding with a sense of purpose to their intended destination. Viewed from above, the foot traffic looks like a river of humanity that ebbs and flows, the single-file streams of people sometimes charging in opposite directions, sometimes merging smoothly in a single headlong rush.

As you make your way along the sidewalk, you notice an obstruction in the flow of people ahead of you. Like a rock in the middle of a river, the obstruction forces the currents of foot traffic to sweep around it.

The obstruction is a man. He's standing in the middle of the sidewalk and he's the only one on the block who's not moving. Like a fighter pilot who has been trained to identify the silhouette of an enemy aircraft from a split-second sighting, you have developed the urban dweller's ability to instantly recognize the spectre confronting you. In one quick glance, you absorb the distinguishing features of an all-too-familiar character. His brown-skinned face is dirty and unshaven. His shaggy black hair is matted and greasy. His clothes are ragged and filthy. One of his eyes is half-open and unfocused, the other is a swollen, purple bruise. He has no front teeth and his drooling mouth is a gaping, twisted hole.

He sways, then lurches and takes two quick steps forward. He jerks his upper body backward to keep from falling on his face. Fighting to keep his balance, he takes a step backwards, then two steps to the side before he resumes a more-or-less stationary swaying stance. His deep voice has a jagged edge and a distinctive accent. As you draw closer he blurts, "Hey! Kin you gimme a quarter?"

By now you've recognized the distinguishing features of this pitiful creature of the urban landscape and made your identification — he's a drunk, a native drunk. He's another drunken Indian.

You've seen him before and you know you'll probably see him again. In spite of his frightening appearance, you can see that he's not dangerous — if you keep moving. But you can also see that the man will be close enough to touch you if you keep walking straight ahead. You are determined not to detour around him and you have no intention of changing direction. Your determination stems from a combination of courage, fear and empathy.

You signal your courage by keeping to your path. After all, you have as much right to the sidewalk as he does and even though he is drunk, dirty and annoying, you're not about to get out of his way.

But part of you is also afraid because you really don't know what he's going to do. You also don't want to be seen as someone who is cowed by a drunken Indian and you are afraid of what others will think if you overreact to this pathetic figure who has done you no harm.

Although he is a repulsive sight, a small measure of empathy stirs within you and makes your pity for him outweigh your disgust. Clearly, he's in bad shape, but you don't want your actions to make him feel worse than he already does, so you keep to your course and try not to make it seem like you're avoiding him. In a curious way, your stick-to-it path expresses your solidarity with downtrodden native people because it shows that you are willing to share the same airspace and the same piece of earth, if only for an instant. But there's a limit to your concern. You don't want him to feel rejected but you also have no intention of giving him what he wants.

So you take a deep breath and grit your teeth. You increase your pace, your heart rate and your blood pressure. You can move past him now in two quick strides and you know that if you don't get by him quickly enough, you'll be inhaling a nau- seating blend of stale liquor and body odour.

You avoid eye contact and stare straight ahead. You can sense him looking at you, waiting for your reply to his request. You won't look at him but you won't look away either. Just as you draw even with the man, you give him your answer — a small, wordless shake of the head. Finally, you take one more stride, pass him and leave him behind.

Two strides later, the tension is lifting from your muscles and you're breathing easier. A block later, the man is no longer in your thoughts. He no longer exists.

Incidents like this play themselves out on Canadian side- walks thousands of times every day and millions of times every year. There's nothing remarkable about these fleet- ing encounters except for one thing: they are one of the few contacts that Canadians have with native people.

Native people, after all, make up less than four percent of Canada's population, and many of them live a world apart from most Canadians — on Indian reserves, in Metis communities and Inuit villages. In addition, many others live a marginalized existence in poor urban neighbour- hoods or are homeless on skid row. Only a tiny fraction of native people have melted into the Canadian mainstream. Most of them, therefore, are invisible to the majority of Canadians.

True, most Canadians "see" native people almost every day. They sit in the same restaurants, ride the same buses and shop in the same stores. On another level, Canadians also "see" native people almost every day in the news media. Native people and native issues are seemingly everywhere. But the perceptions of native people that most Canadians have are defined and limited largely by the second-hand images they see in the media and by the first-hand encounters they have on the street. Given these limited and superficial sources of information, it's not surprising that the stereotype of "the drunken Indian" looms so large in the warped perception that many Canadians have of native people. Although this stereotype is not fully shared by all Canadians, it is nevertheless deeply rooted in the Canadian psyche. In fact, it is as firmly rooted in Canadian belief as is the fairy tale that Europeans settled this land peacefully and without bloodshed.

True, not all Canadians propagate the stereotype, but there's no denying the tremendous impact it has had. There isn't a single native person alive today who has not heard the slur. In fact, it is one of the elements that shapes our lives. At the very least, the stereotype makes native people feel angry, defensive, ashamed or resigned — even if they don't drink. More importantly, the stereotype affects the way others think about us. Ultimately, public attitudes about "drunken Indians" affect government policies about all Indians and all native people.

Although a relatively small but highly visible number of alcoholic misfits have had a disproportionately large impact on the public image of native people, I have not put Crazywater together to downplay or excuse them. Instead, I hope to round out the stereotype — to provide a more complete and accurate understanding of our people's relationship with alcohol.

In doing so, it's tempting to ignore the horrendous aspects of native alcoholism. It's tempting to concentrate solely on people who've quit drinking and on people

who've never drunk in their lives. It's temptir
not very helpful.

There is one basic reason for focusing attention on this
segment of the native population: If people don't understand the native drunk on skid row, they don't understand
the full story of native alcoholism. And if they don't
understand native alcoholism, they don't understand
native people.

On a general level, what should be understood about
native alcoholism is that the stereotype of the drunken
Indian is much more than a dominating and unsightly
phenomenon — it is a symbol of the holocaust that has
wreaked destruction on the Onkwehonwe of Great Turtle
Island for the past three hundred years, and the results
have been horrifying. On an individual level we are paying the legal, medical, financial and social consequences
in the form of beatings, accidents, injuries, suicides, mur-
ders, arrests, jail terms, fires, drownings, sexual abuse,
child abuse, child neglect, poor health, child apprehen-
sions, unemployment and welfare dependency.

But our people have paid an even higher price. We have
lost our languages, medicines and religions. We have lost
our pride, dignity and confidence. We have lost our family values, social patterns and political structures. We have
lost our stewardship over the land. We have lost control
of our lives and our destiny. We have lost almost everything a race of people can lose.

I shudder to think that in my lifetime, by my calcula-
tions, a hundred thousand of my brothers and sisters from
all parts of Great Turtle Island have gone to an early grave
with alcohol in their blood. One hundred thousand! But
they aren't the only ones to go to an early grave. Many
other sober, innocent people have also died because of
native alcoholism. Great Turtle Island moans with the

restless spirits of the victims of a holocaust that has spared no one.

Surveys taken in the Yukon and Saskatchewan show that fully one-third of the adult Indian population has a drinking problem. In Saskatchewan, 38 percent of more than nine hundred adults surveyed said they were either a problem drinker, a chronic drinker or a binge drinker. In the Yukon, 33 percent of the adult Indians surveyed said they were "heavy" drinkers, people who drank more than five drinks on each drinking occasion.

But alcohol abuse affects everyone in the native community. The two-thirds of the community that do not have a drinking problem — the social drinkers, the non-drinkers and the children — still feel the effects, in many different ways, when a friend or family member loses their job, home, family, life or self-respect to alcohol.

If the effects of today's alcoholism are not bad enough by themselves, there is also the reality that every native person alive today is paying the price for the alcoholism of past generations. For example, many of us, maybe even most of us, are survivors of sexual abuse by alcoholic adults. Many of us are dysfunctional adults who are survivors of dysfunctional alcoholic families. And many, especially those of us raised in white foster homes, have lost our identity — we have no idea who we really are; have no idea who we should be; and have no way of becoming the person we should and could have become.

The story of native people and alcohol, then, is appalling. But one of the ironies is that except for a few highly visible people on skid row, native alcoholism is almost invisible. That's because this horrendous problem is felt most deeply in areas that are rarely seen by most Canadians — on Indian reserves, in Inuit villages and Metis communities and on skid row.

One reason why alcoholism is almost invisible is that governments and the media are focusing a lot of attention these days on AIDS — in spite of the fact that alcoholism is, has been, and is likely to be, far more deadly.

The federal government, through Health and Welfare Canada, recognized native alcoholism ten years ago when it established the National Native Alcohol and Drug Abuse Program. In this fiscal year, the department is spending $53 million on the treatment and prevention of native alcoholism and substance abuse. This does not include the government monies spent dealing with the legal, social, economic and medical consequences of native alcoholism.

When I think about the National Native Alcohol and Drug Abuse Program, I can't help thinking that we, as native people, have the dubious distinction of being the only race of people in the country to have a government program geared to combat our alcoholism. Think of it! There are no special programs to deal with other ethnic groups in spite of *their* legendary fondness for beer, wine, vodka, scotch or whiskey. The very existence of the program is a slap in the face. It diminishes our self-esteem by contributing to the misperception that "all native people are drunks."

For its part, the news media pay scant attention to native alcoholism, despite its intrinsic news value and the mounting costs to government and Canadian society. They occasionally report on native alcoholism but usually only when the story involves gory or sensational incidents.

The everyday mundane aspects of this ongoing tragedy are ignored by the mainstream media but native leaders and the native media are just as guilty. For example, native media outlets occasionally report the testimonials of native people who have quit drinking. On these few occasions these people are presented as role models and as positive examples of native sobriety. However, most native media outlets (with few exceptions) deliberately refrain from doing stories about "the problem." As more than one native media executive has told me over the years, "The mainstream news media carry enough bad news about native people. We don't have to do it too."

Like the mainstream news media, the native news media seem to want to downplay or ignore a crisis that directly affects one-third (and indirectly affects the other two-thirds) of the native population. If a third of any other segment of the Canadian population suffered from any other similarly disastrous malady, the outcry and the demand for action would be loud and prolonged — I hope. I'm afraid, though, that we — Canada and its native peoples — have accepted native alcoholism and learned to live with it.

However, as bad as the native media's record is, the record of native political leaders is even worse. For starters, they have a poor record themselves. More importantly, though, they bear the responsibility and they have the opportunity to do something about it.

When it comes to speaking about alcoholism or sobriety, most native leaders are silent, excruciatingly so. Their actions, on the other hand, speak all too loudly. Many native leaders — not most, not all, but many — make obnoxious drunken asses of themselves in public. From time to time some of them pass out in bars, get into drunken brawls, beat their spouses, get caught drunk driving or get arrested for public drunkenness. Given this record, it's no wonder native leaders are so reluctant to condemn alcoholism or promote sobriety. The reason they don't speak out is obvious — they are in the grip of the problem themselves. The fact is that many native leaders at the local, regional and national levels — again, many, not most, not all, but far too many native leaders — have been drunks. These are the very people who are expected to provide leadership, to fight for the people they represent. But it saddens and angers me to realize that more native leaders have probably gone to jail because of drunkenness than because they challenged the law and fought for the rights of their people.

The one positive element in all this is that things used to be worse. Native leaders are now a much more sober lot than they were a generation ago, but sober, non-drinking leaders are still in the minority. Because there are more sober native role models around these days, a generation of young native people may finally grow up to believe that being sober is fashionable and being drunk is foolish, instead of the other way round.

It may seem that I am going out of my way to beat up on native leaders or the native media. I'm not. "White" people and Canadian society bear a huge measure of responsibility for native alcoholism. Although much of this responsibility stems from the past, some of it still rests with the government's continuing refusal to make the necessary changes to allow native people to control their lives and their future.

With few exceptions, individual Canadians are not personally responsible for native alcoholism. One of the exceptions is Gilbert Jordan, a Vancouver barber. Jordan, a white man, was convicted of manslaughter in 1988 and sentenced to prison for poisoning an Indian woman with alcohol. A police investigation found that Jordan bribed and forced the woman to guzzle a large amount of liquor quickly. But she wasn't Jordan's only victim. In the previous eight years, six other native women died of alcohol poisoning after spending a night drinking with him.

To my mind, though, Jordan was just doing on a small scale what Old Man Canada has been doing on a massive scale to native people for the past couple of hundred years. Old Man Canada stripped us of our land, languages, culture, dignity, traditional economies, governments and social structures. Old Man Canada robbed us, raped us and left us with no pride in the past and no hope for the future. Old Man Canada coldly and deliberately poisoned us with his policies and legislation just as surely as if he had held us to the ground with his knee on our chest and used a funnel to pour the booze down our throat.

Are we as native people, then, completely and solely to blame for our alcoholism? No. But it's time we stopped blaming others and started accepting responsibility for changing the situation we're in. The problem of native alcoholism won't be solved until we face up to the problem — as individuals and as a people.

Most people know that the first step in dealing with any addiction is recognizing the problem. While just about everybody in Canada knows about "our problem," many native people are not willing to talk about it openly. So it's up to us as native people to recognize and admit that we have a *huge* drinking problem. That's one of the reasons I decided to do this book. I think *Crazywater* will contribute to this national admission.

We all have stories to tell but not all of our stories are bad. Thousands of native people have turned their lives around. So have a number of entire communities. There are good stories out there, stories of people doing heroic things, stories that need to be shared with the rest of the country. That's another reason I decided to do this book. I hope it will help a few people realize that life can change for the better. I hope it will strengthen our resolve and bind us together. I hope it will help put us on the road to recovery. I hope it will help to start the national healing because the healing must begin. We have to start somewhere, sometime, if we are ever going to get out of the hellhole we're in. That means we're going to have to face up to the truth. Even if it hurts.

Since *Crazywater* is just a partial record of what some of the people I met had to say, it is far from being the last word on the subject of native alcoholism. My only regret is that I could not include more. *Crazywater* does not endorse any of the dozens of theories that have been proposed to explain native alcoholism. Neither does it endorse Alcoholics Anonymous, native spirituality, social drinking or "cold turkey" as the one and only way to deal with native alcoholism. That's because different things work for different people.

Crazywater does stand for something, though. It celebrates sobriety and it celebrates a revival of native culture and traditional spirituality. If I can accomplish just one thing with this book, I hope it is this: I don't want anyone who reads this book ever to walk by a native drunk on the street again without thinking about that person's pain and without thinking about the circumstances that put that person there. I also want people to know that there is much more to the story of native alcoholism — and native sobriety — than just the drunk on skid row. I want people to know that there is a cultural and spiritual revival underway in native communities and it is being inspired and led by sober people. The last thing I want people to know is that despite the devastation we have endured, the Onkwehonwe are going to heal and grow stronger.

1

THE OLD DAYS

"They first tried to get rid of us through disease like smallpox, diphtheria and all that and they couldn't, so they introduced us to this alcohol."

Unlike the peoples of almost everywhere else on Mother Earth, the Onkwehonwe of the northern half of Great Turtle Island did not make or drink alcoholic beverages before Europeans arrived. I like to think that the Onkwehonwe always knew the secret of making alcohol (it's hardly rocket science) but they voluntarily chose not to do so. After all, before the Europeans colonized Great Turtle Island, native people had their pride and their culture intact and they did not have to suffer some of the repressive and depressive elements of contemporary society — things like police and unemployment. As a result, they had no need for the obliterating powers of alcohol.

In any event, the first native hangover on Great Turtle Island no doubt occurred the morning after the first Viking stepped ashore on Newfoundland a thousand years ago. The Onkwehonwe have been on a downhill slide ever since.

17

Alcohol wasn't the only thing the Europeans introduced that had a cataclysmic effect on the Onkwehonwe. Smallpox, measles, malaria, yellow fever and influenza killed from 50 to 90 percent of the Onkwehonwe and paved the way for a European takeover of Great Turtle Island. Although alcohol was not as instantly deadly as the new European diseases, its fatal effects have lasted far longer because unlike the native people's experience with disease, it obviously takes more than a thousand years to build up tolerance or "immunity."

Although it has had a thousand-year history on Great Turtle Island, alcohol's effect on the Onkwehonwe has weakened little with age. Many native people today still undergo an initiation to alcohol that is as shocking and deadly as the first contact must have been ten centuries ago.

The "old days" — the time of native people's first contact with alcohol — linger on in many ways. Many of these first contacts were arranged by fur-traders and whiskey sellers so when native people talk about the old days, many of them burn with resentment or wince with sadness over family and tribal histories scarred by greed and alcohol.

It's not surprising, then, that the awesome power and properties of alcohol have earned it a fearsome reputation and some very descriptive names among the Onkwehonwe.

ISAIAH is a seventy-six-year-old Cree. He lives in Mistissini, a reserve in northern Quebec, four hundred kilometres inland from James Bay. Once husky but now stoop-shouldered, Isaiah is a retired trapper, hunter and fisherman. His story was translated by his son. Isaiah thinks the main event in this story took place about 1886.

In the old days there used to be different trading posts in Quebec. A lot of them are abandoned now but there used to be a trading post here. The main trading post was in Rupert House on the coast of James Bay. It's called Waskaganish now.

The Hudson Bay Company used the best hunters and trappers to do the fur run, to get supplies from Rupert House. My father Johnny was one of those men. These men used to travel down Rupert's River to Waskaganish. They used twenty-four-foot canoes. They took all the pelts that the Bay manager traded that winter and they would bring back supplies. There were over sixty portages. It took about two weeks to go down to the coast and a month to come back up.

And what the men also used to bring back was barrels of whiskey, alcool, I think it was called, 90 percent proof. The Bay used to trade the whiskey with the native people for their fur.

Every year when the men returned from Waskaganish with the liquor the Bay manager would make a party for the whole settlement. He would suppy the food and as much liquor as you could drink. The whole town would be drunk for the night.

Then one year the post manager in Waskaganish told my father and the other men that there was a law prohibiting liquor to be sold to Indians. So instead of going up the rivers with their usual load of booze, they went back with just flour, tea and lard. When the canoe brigade got to Mistissini, all the villagers and the Bay manager came to meet them. Solomon Voyageur, the captain of the canoe brigade, told the Bay manager, "We didn't bring an ounce of liquor. We brought good stuff — food for the native people. We have flour, tea and lard and not an ounce of liquor."

And of course, everybody in Mistissini was looking forward to the annual *bash*. When they heard that there was gonna be no party that summer, a lot of the old men and old ladies in the community cried. I guess they were really sad there wouldn't be a party that year.

My dad used to always tell me that story and laugh about it. My father never drank, eh? And he often wondered why people would cry. Like you cry if somebody passes away and all that, but you don't cry because there's not gonna be a party. But they did.

MARINE is a short, wiry-haired, fifty-two-year-old grandmother from a reserve in southern Alberta.

Alcohol was introduced into our community in my great-grandfather's time because I remember my grandparents telling us the time when they were trading whiskey with fur. They were living up Nordegg way and my grandmother said they used to trade horses and fur at Rocky Mountain House, I think it was. She used to tell us about this story that my great-grandmother was addicted to it and she was crying for more whiskey.

So my great-grandfather had to sell this one last horse for a barrel of whiskey. So he went there and all this time my great-grandmother was crying for the whiskey. My great-grandfather went on the horse, traded that horse for whiskey and he rolled that whiskey barrel I don't know how many days. He rolled it back to where they were living.

My grandmother used to tell me this story. That whiskey barrel we used after for a water barrel. My mother remembers that story too.

The white people just manipulated us so they could get

rid of us so they could have all the land, eh? They first tried to get rid of us through disease like smallpox, diphtheria and all that and they couldn't, so they introduced us to this alcohol.

REG is a tall, folksy and thoughtful Cayuga elder. He is sixty-eight years old and is a leader of the traditional Longhouse religion on the Six Nations Grand River Territory in southern Ontario. Some of the people there believe they can protect themselves from witches in the community by pouring alcohol across their doorways and window sills to keep out the witchcraft. Reg began the interview by commenting on that belief.

There's people that believe, "I'll have a little drink and protect me so nobody can witch me." It makes sense because the witch medicine, love medicine or whatever, is made from Indian medicine — roots, plants and so on. One of the taboos is that you can't drink alcohol while you're taking Indian medicine or you'll kill that medicine. Alcohol will kill any medicine so that's why they do that, to kill any medicine that's used against them. That's why they use it for protection, some of them. If you're taking medicine for any reason, like you're taking medicine for cancer or any kind of sickness, you can't drink because it's common knowledge that that kills the medicine.

Alcohol will kill medicine because it's evil. Alcohol's an evil thing, you see, it's not ours. The Creator gave it to our white brothers to give them new strength at the end of the day when he's working hard. He's allowed three drinks a day, a white man, because he's got so much work it makes him feel better. He's allowed three and we are not allowed any at all because we don't live the same as the white man.

A person must not drink at all. These are Longhouse people I'm talking about. No drinking at all. Not a drop. That's our belief. It's not for us.

ROSEMARIE is a forty-nine-year-old Ojibway who lives in Toronto and works for the Government of Ontario. She quit drinking seventeen years ago.

I asked my mother before she died what the word was for "drunk" in Ojibway and she said, *geeshkwaybee.* I asked her to translate that literally in English as to how she understood what she was saying and *geeshkwaybee* was "crazy-in-the-head." I thought that was really appropriate.

DESCENDING CLOUD is a soft-spoken seventy-year-old Cayuga man from the Grand River Territory in southern Ontario.

The old people used to call it "poison water." Sometimes they called it "firewater" because it burns, it starts on fire. Now, the word is the same in all the Iroquois languages. In Mohawk they call it *deganigohadaynyohs* — it changes the mind, "the mind-changer." They call it that because the native people did not have alcohol before the Europeans came here to Turtle Island.

The story goes that the first time the native people used it was from the fur-traders. When the native people traded pelts and furs, they got alcohol by the keg.

When they tasted it they began wondering why their mind began to change — they never felt like that before. They were not in their right minds, it made them laugh and stagger around. It was powerful in how it changed the mind of a person, it affected your mind. It was very powerful.

LAZARUS is a smiling, barrel-chested seventy-four-year-old Stoney from southern Alberta.

Alcohol is *gahtonejabee meenee*. *Gahtonejabee*, that's the Stoney word for "drunk." *Meenee* means "water." So it means "crazy water," the water that makes you go crazy.

PATRICIA is a fifty-year-old Ojibway who grew up in northern Ontario.

There's different names for it, like for alcohol, the real alcohol with a lot of fire in it, we used to call it "firewater" — *skwidayabo*.

I used to see my parents make moonshine. First they had to make homebrew with yeast, sugar, bran and they put some kind of fruit in it — raisins or prunes or oranges and warm water. They used to call it *neboop* — it just meant "mixture." In a day or so you have your homebrew ready to drink. And once it sets, they would use their distiller and boil it over slow heat. There's a little spout at the end of the distiller and that's where the moonshine would come out. When the first drop came out, they would put it in a spoon and light a match and that spoon would catch fire. That's how they knew it was a powerful drink and that's why they called it firewater.

SUMMERCLOUDS *is a forty-six-year-old Ojibway man from a reserve on Georgian Bay in south central Ontario.*

What we called it was *shkode-waabo. Shkode* is fire; *waabo* is water — firewater. That was the word for hard liquor or moonshine. Like when they drank it, it was just like fire going down their throat. This is the way they described it.

The proper word for wine would be *zhiim-nabo*. It means something that is made from grapes. That is the correct terminology but the slang and more definite word is *giiwnaadzi-waabo* and when you put it in English, it's crazywater. *(laughs)* They called it that because wine has the potential to really make people just drunk right out of their mind, I guess. People act really abnormal because of it. They get falling down drunk and say crazy things; it's like a person is crazy or possessed. People knew what they were talking about.

HAROLD *is a thirty-eight-year-old Carrier from the Necoslie Band in central British Columbia.*

Nedotou, they call it. In our language that's the word for liquor. *Nedo* means "white man" and *tou* means "water," so it's "white man's water." It was only the white people used to be allowed to drink at one time, so that's why they called it that because only white people were allowed to buy it.

MILLIE *is a round-faced thirty-four-year-old inuk. She is short and perky, and gestures often with her hands.*

Imialuk covers all the alcoholic beverages. *Imi* is water, *aluk* is bad — "bad water." When somebody drank, it turned them bad. Like when my people found out what it does to other people who had been drinking, that's how it got its name. If you drink it, it turns you bad.

🥀

JULIA *is a thin, withered eighty-year-old Alberta Cree with a lively sense of humour. She has never drunk in her life. Her comments were translated by her daughter.*

When I was seventeen years old, I start to learn Indian medicine. My dad teach me. When I first start studying them roots, these two elders came to me. They called me on up to the house. My dad take me over. He telled me, "Those people, they're going to pray."

I told him, "No. I don't want to go."

"Let's go."

So I went over and they put nice blanket and they seat me in the middle. Those people they standing and singing Indian song. And dance. I was so scared. They pray for me. "You going to be medicine woman."

Ever since I was blessed by these elder people, I never drink or do anything because they told me that I'm gonna be like a witch doctor in the future for the young generation to come. That's why I never drink a day.

I know that kind of medicine. My older son quit drinking by Indian medicine. My son was so bad when he gets drunk. He drink everything. He loved to drink. He used to come around and threatened us so each evening we had to stay outside until he goes away. We were always hiding outside from him. And I didn't like that so I go and made up prescription. I used the medicine. You have to make like a tea, eh? The medicine is from the roots. They're hard to get. We have to go down to the States, B.C., Hobbema, Saddle Lake at this time of the year. We have to pick the ripe one out. We all sit and clean them, dry and pack them up. Sometimes my daughter put in the jar.

I know prescription but I don't tell anyone.

One time after he was finished drinking, he came to the house and that's the time. He wants tea and I gave it to him without letting him know. I gives medicine that makes him don't like it. He go outside, he throw up. Cleaned that blood out. (*laughs*) He thinks there's something trouble in his stomach. (*laughs*) He said, "Oh Mom, your food is not good." (*laughs*) That's what he said.

That's how he quit. He just thrown up. Quit. Right away. He doesn't know. Just like tea, you know. I just give without asking. (*laughs*) He never drink after that. He was about twenty-three years old. He's just about sixty now and I been watching him after that. He still doesn't know. If we tell him he might get mad. So I never tell him. (*laughs*)

I have another boy too. I gave him that too. Young boy. He doesn't drink anymore. Before he used to have a fighting, eh? Terrible. He's been sober for many years now. He quiet down kind of nice. He got married and he has little girl. He working right now. He doesn't care about drinking. That's the only other one I done. I don't bother other people. I don't do to anybody else. Nobody. Just those two boys. No one knows about it. Just myself and my daughter.

🌀

THERESA'S STORY

Theresa is a well-dressed, vibrant and attractive forty-one-year-old Dogrib with high cheekbones and wide, sparkling eyes. She has a distinctive accent that causes her to pronounce "happy" as "habby." She underwent treatment for alcoholism six times before she finally quit drinking nine years ago. She is now an addictions counsellor in Yellowknife.

I was raise up in Fort Rae, jus' a small little settlement in the Northwest Territories. I grew up in a home where there was no alcohol involved. I never did see too much of people drinkin' at all until when I got married in 1968.

I marry a guy from Fort Providence. I married when I was seventeen. We moved to Fort Providence and that was when I started to notice people drinkin' there. I was askin' some people question, like, "Why are these people so habby all the time? Why are they laughin' and jokin' and yelling?"

That's when I realized, "So this is what happens to people when they drink!" You know? They feel much habbier and much excited and have lot of fun.

So when we were livin' in Fort Providence, that was in 1970, that's when my firs' time that I had ever tase the booze was. My husband took me out to the bar and I joined the crowd and have the firs' tase of my beer. It tase awful but the more I see people laughin' and jokin' and dancin', I thought, "*Whoa.* I'm gonna be like them person. It's okay if this beer tase awful. I'll jus' drink it anyway."

I had my firs' beer and then I had my second beer and then that's when I black out. I don't remember anything. And the next day when I woke up I was jus' really sick.

But at that time I didn't know that the sick that I had was a hangover. I thought that maybe I was sick from the flu. So I went to the hospital and I went to see the nurse and I tol' her I was really sick. I said my head was really painful and my stomach was really upset and I want to puke and everything. And she burs' out laughing at me (*laughs*) and she said, "You ever know that when people drink, the next day they're sick?"

And I says, "No. This is the firs' time I ever tase the alcohol." But I said, "Gee, I had fun las' night but today I sure in the hell don't feel like havin' fun at all."

And she said, "Do you ever heard 'bout a hangover?"

And I said, "A hangover?" To *me*, I thought a hangover means you're hang over something, like a steel bar or something. So I said, "Is there anything you can give me for my hangover?"

And she says, "No. There's nothing for that. You jus' have to suffer with it."

So I went home and my husband started laughin' at me and he says, "The only way that you're going to cure the hangover is by goin' back to the bar and have another couple of beers and the hangover will go away."

So when I went back to the bar they tol' me I was barred out and I said, "Sheesus. What did I do?"

They tol' me, "You're not allowed to come back in the bar."

I jus' couldn't *believe* it. They said I was barred out for ninety-nine years. (*laughs*) Hones'! So I musta really done something. (*laughs*)

That was my firs' time. But after I got used to it, the booze really did tase good for me. And I used to get into really heavy drinking. I used to drink hard stuff and use the beer as a chaser instead of using water. I used to drink navy rum and I would mix it with Coke. If there's no Coke, then I use water. If there's no water, I use tea or coffee. *Anything* with it. (*laughs*) It doesn't matter how it tase. I didn't give a damn.

And I also use to tas' homemade brew too. *God*, you drink that homemade brew, raisin floats in your mouth, *ptoo-ptoo*, jus' spit out the raisin. (*laughs*)

So ever since then I was drinkin' like maybe 'bout two or three times a month. I was drinkin' only if my husband gives me a permission. Then I go out drinkin' with him. If not, then I'm to stay home and look after the house. And I drink until I get my blackouts. I don't remember anything and when I come to, I would be up with either a shiner, a black eye or swelling lips or can't even barely walk. And I tell my husband, "What happened?"

He said, "Nothing."

So I said, "Who did these to me? Who beat me up?"

And he says, "You. You fall down."

But then I found out from other people that he beat me up but I didn't remember because I black out. So I guess when I drink and the alcohol takes a control of me, I do all these foolish things — like maybe talkin' to people that I wasn't supposed to talk to. Or saying something that I'm not supposed to say. Or maybe laugh or smile at another person that I'm not supposed to. So my husband beat me up for that.

But at that time I thought, "Oh, okay. So this is life. That's the way it's supposed to be. He's got the rights to do whatever he wants with me. He can beat me up, he can push me around because he's my husband." That's the way I was raised up, so that's the way I look at it.

It was going on like that till 1972. My husband got a job offering in Edzo as a heavy-duty equipment operator. So we moved to Edzo and that's when we got a place of our own and I thought, "Now here we are — livin' by ourself and things are gonna change. He's gonna slow down his drinkin' and things will be so beautiful." Like the way I always been dreaming about.

But the more we were livin' alone in Edzo the worse the drinkin' continued. Like him and I were both drinkin' almos' every, every, every weekend for four years. But he was abusin' me a lot and I was really afraid of him.

I remember so many times that I tried to quit drinkin' because my parents said, "Alcohol are only for a man. It's not for a woman. Woman are not allowed to drink. Woman are allowed to stay home and look after their house and look after their kids."

So I never bothered drinkin' and he did. He comes home and then he get mad at me. Like he tells me that I was out someplace and I wasn't doin' the cookin', I wasn't cleaning up the house. And I thought, *"Gee,* you know, when I was drinkin' I never hear these nasty words. I never hear him complaining. When I'm tryin' to sober up, he doesn't seem to be habby about it. What does he want?"

So I started to join him again. I started to drink every weekend until 1974. I was working in Edzo hospital and I was a housekeeper. That kep' me sober because I sometime hadda work on the weekend. Then when I come home I find out that my husband's gone out to Yellowknife and I know exackly what's gonna happen when he come home. Like he's gonna start arguin' with me, he's gonna start fightin' me. So what I usually do was tell the kids, "We're gonna stay over at Gramma's."

And that's the way it was every weekend. I was running away from home. I was going to Fort Rae, staying over at my mum and dad. Jus' protecting myself from gettin' beat up and getting a licking for no reason.

The only person that he abused a lot was jus' me. He never lay hand on the kids. Jus' me. I was gettin' beaten up and so I thought, "He never lays hands on the kids, so I might as well jus' leave the kids and run away and come back later when he pass out."

I never did have a really good home 'cause of alcohol. We never had a real good Christmas together. Christmas is the day for him to get drunk. I'm forgotten. The kids are forgotten. They didn't know anything about Christmas trees, Christmas presents, nothing like that.

And then I los' interest in my job and I started to negleck my kids. Like the alcohol was so important to me that I sometime didn't care whether they have food or they don't have food, whether they have a sitter or they don't have a sitter. Sometime when I come home after gettin' on a big drunk for two, three days I find out the house is empty, the kids are gone and my husband's still out someplace drinkin' and the firs' thing is I run around lookin' for my kids. Then I find out that the social service took my kids. Through alcohol the social service has been takin' my kids away from me at leas' three to four times.

One night when my husband was still beatin' me up, the RCMP they walk in and they took him and throw him in jail. And then the RCMP, he tol' me this abusing has been going on and on and on. He says, "It's only up to *you* to stop that. *You* have to stop this."

But I said, "*How* am I supposed to stop this? I tried everything. I run away from home so many time to teach him a lesson to tell him that I'll come back to you only after you quit beatin' me up."

He said, "The abusin' has to stop. You've been landing in the hospital. You've been running away from home. Social service has been taking your kids. If only your husband lef' you alone, things would change."

So I said, "Well, okay, where can I go?"

So he says my husband's goin' to court next week. "At that time I expeck you to go to court. And then there's a name there, it's called legal separation. You ever heard about it?"

I said, "No." Everything was so new to me. I never heard of that.

So anyway we went to court a week after. I didn't have to say much because the RCMP were doing mos' of the work for me and the public health nurse and the social service were involved too.

So all three of them got together. They tol' the jury my story so all I had to say was I wanted a peace bond so he doesn't have to hurt me again and he doesn't have to go near the kids.

So they allowed that. We were separated for a year but during that time I realized that while I was livin' alone I was *really* drinkin' heavy and I was really negleckin' my kids. Like I was coming to Yellowknife every weekend. I never come home.

I was still workin' at the hospital and then one day my boss tol' me, he said, "Theresa, you gotta do something 'bout your drinkin'. You're drinkin' too much. You're gonna lose your job if you don't smarten up." And then he said, "You ever heard about Alcohol Anonymous?"

And I said, "Alcohol Anonymous? What's the Alcohol Anonymous?"

He said Alcohol Anonymous is a place for people to sober up. And I said, "No, I hadn't heard about it. What does it do to people? And where do you go for that?"

And he says there's a treatment centre named "detox" in Yellowknife that you can go to.

So I said, "If I go, will I still hang onto my job?" You see I was thinking if he say "no," then I'll say, "The hell with it. I'm not gonna go."

But he say, "Yes. Your job will be still waiting for you when you get back."

I said, "How 'bout my kids? How 'bout my home?"

"Don't worry about these things. We'll handle them."

So I said, "Okay, I'll go."

The firs' time I ever stepped foot in the detox, I was really scared, nervous, shy. And also I was really angry of the people. "Why do they have to bring me in here for?"

I was thinking to myself that this is no place for me. I have to be home with my kids. My kids need me. But I jus' thought, "Well, I give a try and see if it's gonna work for me. If it works for other people, maybe it'll work for me."

So I was in the detox for my twenty-eight days program. And after I finished my program, I phoned home. I found out social service again took the kids away.

And this time I thought, "*Now* what?" You know? "Here I am, I'm tryin' to sober up. Why have they took my kids away?"

So I went right back in the bar and started drinkin' again. When I firs' took my program, I wasn't really doin' it for myself. I was doin' it for my job. I was doin' it for my family. I was doin' it for my kids. I did it for other people. I wasn't doin' it for *me*. I didn't want to quit drinkin'. I wanted to continue drinkin'.

So I did. I went right back to alcohol again. I was livin' in Yellowknife. I was jus' drinkin' steady, steady, steady. Then my boss somehow got hol' of me and he tol' me, "You're not getting anywhere."

So I said, "Is there any other detox beside Yellowknife? Is there any other places where I can go? I know so many people on the street that every time I leave from here I drink."

Here I am blamin' other people again. It's the people's fault. It's not my fault.

So he says, "You ever heard about Bonneyville in Alberta?"

"No."

"Well," he said, "They have another rehab centre there and if you really want to go, you can."

So I lef' to Bonneyville. That was the same year, in '75. I took another twenty-eight days program in Bonneyville, then I moved back to Rae and got my job back and got my kids back. Got my home. I didn't go back to my husband.

And I stay sober for three months. Then I start drinkin' for, oh, 'bout three years, I think. And then I came back here again to this detox centre and I took another twenty-eight days program. That was my third time.

After a year my husband and I got back together. We were really drinking a lot but he quit hitting me around. He got his job back and I was still working at the hospital, so we have money coming to us. Like we make sure there was groceries for the kids. We make sure that we had a good babysitter before we come to Yellowknife.

At that time, liquor wasn't allowed in Rae, so we got caught so many time. He had so many fine to pay because of gettin' caught with booze. Or else drinkin', driving.

And then finally in 1982, his mother was really, really sick. So she call us. She was at the Hay River hospital.

I remember that the elders used to say to me, "When a person is close to dying, remember what was the las' message that they gave you and it will do you good for the res' of your life."

All these years that I was drinkin', she was doin' the babysittin'. She was the mother to my kids. So we went to visit her. She asked for me, so I went and sat with her. She said, "The only thing I'm worryin' about is my grandchild. If I die, who's gonna look after them? Who's gonna feed them? Who's gonna dress them up and send them to school?"

So I look at her and I said, "Well, I'm the mother. I could do those things."

She say, "You never did because you were too busy drinkin'." She grab hol' of my hand and she said, "Can I ask a favour from you?"

And I said, "Sure, what is it?"

She said, "Would you please quit drinkin'?"

And I said, "Well, how 'bout your son? Why me? If your son quit drinkin', I will too."

And she said, "My son is my son but it's you I'm worryin' about. I want you to quit so you can look after the kids. You were doin' real good before and I'm sure you can do that again."

So I tol' her, "I'm not gonna promise you that I will. But I will try."

I don't know whether my husband listen to what the mother said but that night when we got back to our hotel room, we had three bottles of twenty-six ounces in our hotel room. He took those bottles and he poured it down the toilet bowl. He said, "That's it. We're not gonna drink again anymore."

And I wanted so much for him to sober up, so I said, "Are you sure?"

And he said, "Yeah, I'm sure."

But I said, "You know we can't do it on our own. We gotta have a support. We gotta have something to help us to quit drinking."

So we both took the twenty-eight days program. But it was really hard for me because my husband was a really jealous person. I couldn't dare explain my feelings or share what I really wanted to share about how my life was and how it was when I was drinkin' because I was really scared of what he's gonna say to me after.

So we both stayed sober through '82, '83 and '84. I started AA meetings and women's support group meetings in Rae. I used to put up a poster saying, "There's a AA meeting tonight at this time, at this place. Please be there if you need help."

For a whole year I was goin' to Fort Rae, goin' into the friendship centre, make coffee, lay AA pamphlets, have AA books, having the door open. You know. But for a whole year I was goin' to meeting all by myself. And I was really angry (*laughs*) 'cause I wanted to sober up the whole town. Because I was sober, I expeck everybody to sober up. You know. I wanted to help the people so bad.

But through the one year of my sobriety I wasn't really workin' on my program because I have so much to do. Like I was really hyper. I was always on the go, go, go. I was cleaning up the house. I was running to work. I go home, laundry.

Since we sober up we had a new truck. We bought new furnitures. I started to keep my place clean. We fix up the house and the kids were doing good. Like everything was jus' workin' so good. Like we had this couple friend of ours. They see us being sober and they see us being habby, the kids are habby, that even them, they sober up. And we thought, "Well, *there*. At leas' we have somebody, a friend of ours, that are sober."

And then what I did was I switch my sobriety around to gambling. Instead of goin' to AA meeting, I started goin' to bingos. I started playing cards every night. I *hadda* go to the bingo. I *hadda* go to Rae to play cards 'cause if I don't go one day, I get mad at my husband, I get mad at my kids.

And my mum was telling me, "You gonna lose. You gonna go back drinkin'."

I said, "No, I'm not. When you go to bingo, there's nobody drinkin' there. When you go to card game, there's nobody drinkin' there. So I won't go back drinkin'."

So after my three years of being sober, I got a call from the detox saying if I want to come back to take my two weeks' follow-up. So I said, "Sure, I needed that."

So my husband and I came back to the detox. That's when one of the counsellor tol' me, "Theresa you have to quit that bingo. You have to quit that gambling because it's another addiction."

At that time I still have resentful towards her because she sober me up and I said, "You don't know anything. All you know is how to sober up people. Don't you tell me to quit bingo. The more important thing in this world is at leas' I'm not drinkin'. I lef' that disease. Bingo has nothing to do with alcohol."

I used to hate her. I used to always get mad at her and tell her to get out of my back. "I'll do whatever *I* want. *Nobody* has the right to tell me what to do. No one. I sober up. From now on nobody's gonna control me."

But after our follow-up, he went back drinkin' and I stayed sober. I quit bingo. I give up playing cards. And I couldn't really cope with it. I tol' him, "If you want to drink, you stay away from home."

But then I found out he was involved with another lady and every time that he was with her, he was drinkin'. And that really, really hurt my feelings. I said, "Here I am, I'm being sober. I'm a nice woman. I'm not drinkin'. I'm not goin' to bingo. I'm not gonna play cards."

I was nagging him. I was yelling at him. I was calling him down. And I even threat him. "If you're not gonna quit drinkin', I'm gonna kill myself."

And then I blame the social service, blame the RCMP, blame the doctor, blame the pries', blame everybody in

Fort Rae. It's everybody's fault. It's not my fault. So what I did was I jus' isolated myself. I quit goin' to the meetings. I jus' lock my doors. Shut my curtains. Jus' stay home.

I was like that for one whole month until in '85, I went to Poundmaker to take my two weeks' follow-up. I went alone. I was still sober then, but I wasn't working my program.

They decided to keep me for twenty-eight days. So I said, "Okay, sure." So after I finished my twenty-eight days program, they decide to keep me for my two weeks' follow-up. And so I stay in Poundmaker for six weeks.

That's where I started to understand. I started to learn what relapse is and what gambling does to people. People can get into all kinds of addiction after they sober up. I was on my dry drunk. I learn so many things when I was in Poundmaker.

And then they also help me to learn to change my life around. Like I was not to enable my husband anymore. I was not to nag at him anymore. *He* has to make his own choice. *He* has to do whatever is good for him. Because I'm sober doesn't mean that I can sober up everybody.

When I came back to Yellowknife I really changed around. I didn't nag at him about anything, I jus' let him be. I was always enabling him. I was always making phone calls for him. I was always running around for cigarette for him. Running around and baby him and do so many things for him. So when I came back from Poundmaker, I changed that around.

One day in 1986, two weeks before Christmas, I went home on Monday because I thought, "Oh, he'll be at work." I went home and here he was sleeping. I went in the bedroom and I woke him up and I said, "Aren't you supposed to be at work?"

And he said, "Yeah, but I'm sick. Could you make a phone call for me? Phone my boss and tell my boss I can't make it 'cause I'm too sick."

And I said, "No. I'm not makin' no phone calls for you. If *you* wanna phone, you phone. I'm not doin' it."

So he hit me on the face and I hit him back. I was really surprised. I was gonna say, "I'm sorry, I didn't mean to hit you." But I thought, "I don't need to apologize. He hit me, I get right back."

I said, "All these years I live with you, I been hittin' around, being threat by you. This time I'm sober and all I was waiting for was for you to hit me. *That's it.* I don't need to be hitten around anymore."

And then I said, "Either you leave or I'll leave. I don't want my kids to grow up in a home like this anymore. They have been for nineteen years living with you. They have been brought up in abusing home. They see you beat me up. They see you and I drinkin'. They grew up sometimes there was no food for them to eat. Sometime they have no place to go. It's not gonna happen again. Not ever again."

So I called the RCMP because at that time, in 1986, that's when I learned that if a man starts slappin' or hittin' their wife or their woman around, they can get charged for that. So I thought, "I'm gonna charge him," 'cause so many times in the pas' years I charge him and I drop it off or else I don't even show in court. But this time I says, "I'm doin' it."

So I phoned the RCMP, and the RCMP came over and I tol' them what happen. I say, "He punch me on my face." My face was all swelling up and bruises.

So the RCMP said, "Could we bring you someplace where it's nice and safe?"

So then I thought of this lady in Rae. "Could you bring me down to her place? I'm gonna live with her for a while."

So they brought all my stuff over and I lef' the kids with their dad because the kids are ol' enough now and he never does lay hand on them. He might yell and scol' and swear at them and that was it. So they stayed with their dad.

I stay with her for a week. I tol' her what I was going through and she said, "You ever heard about Alison McAteer House in Yellowknife?"

And I said, "What is it?" *Again* there was something new to me.

She said, "It's a place where women go for support from gettin' beaten up from your husband. I'm sure you can go there. That would be a good place for you to go."

I said, "Is that another detox?" But I was jus' joking.

So anyway they phoned and two days later, social service came and pick me up and my two younges' son and they brought us to Alison McAteer House. They welcome us in there. But I was really scared when I firs' got in there. I thought, "Gee. What are they gonna do with me now?"

I was really lonely, homesick. I wanted to be back at home with my people. I always have in my mind that, "Someday I'm gonna help my people. Someday I'm gonna do something for them."

So I stay in Alison McAteer House for a whole month. My two younges' son were living there with me too. And my kids were going to family counsellor meetings 'cause they needed that.

In 1987, I got a job there working with battered women, counselling. I work there for a year and nine months. I took so many workshops. I know I did a lot of my personal growth. And then in 1989, the executive of Northern Addictions Service call me and she says, "Do you know that we have an opening at the detox centre?"

So I stop at her office and I pick up the application. This was something new for me, like I'm not well educated. I only went as far as to grade six. The next day I got interviewed at eleven o'clock in the morning. By twelve o'clock I was hired. (*laughs*) And I said, "*Whoa*. That was *easy*." You know. Because I never went through these kind of things.

I said, "*Jesus Chris'*, here I am. I dress up so good and I thought you guys were gonna complain about the way I was dress and the way I was talking."

She said, "No. We like the way you are. The main important thing is you got the feel, you got the experiences. You got everything."

When they tol' me, I was lookin' around. I said, "What do I got? I don't know what I got."

See how we don't look at ourself? I learn from other people. When other people tell me something, I said, "*Oh*, so that's the way I am." But I never get a chance to have a good look at myself because all these years people were always putting me down.

Like when I used to get beat up from my husband or from my mum and dad, I used to think, "Okay, that was my mistake. I have to go and say I'm sorry for what I did. It was my fault. I didn't meant to do that."

For *all* these years I was carrying that. So when I got a job offering I sat there and I said, "Really?"

She said, "You're a nice person."

I said, "Really?" I didn't know. All these times I was always puttin' myself down. Everything was no good about me. 'Cause I heard it so many times that I jus' couldn't seem to let go of it. But then finally goin' to AA meeting really helped me a lot.

One thing I found out living in Yellowknife there was a lot of AA members. I was goin' to AA meetings every, every, every night 'cause I know I need it. I was going to family counsellors. I was going to battered women meeting. I was going to *so many* meetings. The meetings were jus' coming out of one ear to another ear. But I realized that the only thing that really help me was the AA. My fellowship really helped me to stay sober.

I'm starting to understand. I'm starting to learn. I'm starting to feel *different*. I really changed. A lot of people in my home town, they seen that. So many things about me that they see, they jus' couldn't believe.

I've been sober for nine years. And since 1989 I've been working in this kind of a field, here in the detox.

My husband's been sober for the las' three and a half months now. I don't have any resentful towards him. I tol' him, "I'm not livin' with you now and you're not goin' to hit me so I might as well throw my garbage at you." (*laughs*) So he jus' laugh at me. Now we're jus' the bes' of friends. Through AA I learned not to hate him.

All these things that happened to me was on account of jus' one lousy thing, was the alcohol. Now that I lef' it alone, I'm another different person. I'm my own self. I can smile. I can laugh. I can talk with anybody I want. I got my own bank account. I know how to budget my money. I can go wherever I want to go. I don't have to worry 'bout anything. I don't have to come home and say, "Oh shit. Now I have to face this miserable person."

I got my spirituality back. I pray all the time. That is my ol' tradition. I got that back. I go hunting. I go fishing. I go trapping and I still sew.

Now I'm really habby. I got a good home, a good job, a good person. I guess I can call him my husband 'cause I've been living with him for over a year now, a real understanding person. I got a guy that always remind me, "I love you."

I realize I was a people pleaser. I was always doing things for other people 'cause I want them to love me because my parents never did love me. My husband never did love me. The only time he say he love me was only after he beats me up. I ask him, "Why you do that?"

"Because I love you."

Same with my parents. "Why you hit me for?"

"Because we love you. Because we want you to grow up the right way." (*laughs*) Am I supposed to grow up the right way when I get beat up all the time?

The program and the AA meeting really help me a lot. I work my program really good and it really helps.

I remember when I firs' sober up, I want everything to work for me. I wanna have a good home, good kids, a good job. I want everybody to sober up. Now, I don't need to have that. The main important thing to me now is that as long as *I'm* the one that's sober, that's okay. I'm learning to forgive and forget about my past.

And now I feel really habby and thankful for the things that I have went through because now I can help other people. It was a painful journey but now I got something back for it. Like now I finally got what I want.

I look up and say, "Why *me*?" You know? "Why *me*? I hurt so many people. I negleck my kids. I done so many bad things. Why am I getting everything that I always wanted?"

But then I sometime think it's because I been working really, really hard for the las' nine years. My higher power mus' have give me a reward 'cause now I help a lot of people. Right now, boy, things are jus' workin' so good for me. I'm so habby that my husband is staying sober and all my boys are doing really good.

So — habby ending. (*laughs*) I sometime can't believe it.

2

Prohibition

"When somebody bought a bottle of wine, you don't want the police to find you with that open bottle because you're gonna get fined or you're gonna go to jail."

In 1868, the year following Confederation, Parliament passed the first *Indian Act*. One of its provisions made it illegal for status Indians to buy or possess alcohol. Indian prohibition lasted 117 years and was not entirely abolished until 1985. Thousands of Indian people were arrested and jailed as a result of this law, many of them dozens of times. The law against Indian drinking was not added to the books just to appease churches or temperance groups. It was a convenient social control measure that could be arbitrarily used by Indian agents and the police against whomever they wanted to target.

Of course the law didn't stop or prevent Indians from drinking, but it did change the way they drank — for the worse. Since Indians were forbidden to buy liquor, they frequently resorted to drinking other far more dangerous intoxicants. The law also reinforced a destructive drinking culture that Indian people evolved after their first contacts with hard-drinking soldiers and scheming fur-traders. Since they were not allowed in bars or taverns and since they were not permitted to possess alcohol in their homes, the law forced them to become furtive and drink in bushes and back alleys. More ominously, Indians also had to guzzle their beer, wine or liquor as quickly as possible to keep from being arrested.

To legally gain the right to drink and vote, Indians had to sign away their rights and "enfranchise" themselves. In legal terms, this meant that they became full Canadian citizens. In the eyes of most Indians, however, they became "white."

It should be remembered that until twenty years ago, the stated goal of Canada's native affairs policy was to extinguish Indian and aboriginal rights and to assimilate Indian people into mainstream society and turn them into "little brown Canadians." One of the methods the federal government used to achieve this goal was to enact the prohibition and enfranchisement provisions of the *Indian Act*. Together with the prohibition against Indian drinking, the enfranchisement provisions were extremely damaging because they helped split "Indian country" into "status" and "non-status" factions. That rift continues to exist and may never be healed.

During World War II, thousands of Indian men joined the military, where they gained the right to drink legally. Once they left the army and returned home, however, they were once more prohibited from drinking by the *Indian Act*. In the generation following the war, the ban on Indian drinking in towns and cities began to fade. Indians gradually gained the right to buy and possess alcohol in different jurisdictions by the mid-1960s.

Finally, the *Indian Act* provision that prohibited Indians from buying or possessing alcohol "in town," was struck down by a Supreme Court of Canada ruling in 1970. But on reserves, Indians continued to be prohibited from possessing alcohol unless the reserve's band council specifically voted to allow it. Since 1985, that situation has been reversed, so that Indian reserves are all now automatically "wet" unless a band council specifically votes to make it "dry." Of six hundred local Indian governments across the country, almost two hundred have voted themselves dry since 1985.

ELIZABETH is a strong-willed, middle-aged Blood who learned a lot of local history from her ninety-seven-year-old grandmother.

Back then there was no drinking because this was a dry reserve. There was very, very little drinking. The crime rate on this reserve at that time was nil, almost nil. If somebody was drinking and it got out into the community, you know, "So-and-so was drinking," that family was shamed. It was really looked down on, drinking was.

Going way back to the 1930s and 1920s, the Indian agent was just like a God on this reserve. The Indian agent dictated our lives and if he found out that someone had been drinking over a month ago, even through rumour, he would ride out to that person's place and tell them, "You were drunk one month ago. Now you will pay me five dollars."

And five dollars back then was a lot of money. That happened to lots of people back then. But once they opened the liquor stores and the bars and licensed premises to the Indian people here, I just saw a total change almost overnight. It was just totally unreal. Fights day in and day out, and that's when a lot of young people died.

There was so much hatred and so much animosity between the Indians and the whites in the surrounding towns. There's a lot of prejudice, eh? After a few years the drinking started to taper off, but the white people still stereotype everyone as a drunk.

KATE is a large, slow-moving sixty-three-year-old grandmother. Before she quit drinking twenty-six years ago, she was given twenty-two separate jail terms for drunkenness, not counting the number of times she was held overnight in the drunk tank and released the next day without being charged. All of her arrests were for violations of the Indian Act *prohibition. She is now an addictions counsellor in Alberta.*

When it was against the law for Indians to drink, that's where it all started, this drinking going out of control, 'cause when somebody bought a bottle of wine, you don't want the police to find you with that open bottle because you're gonna get fined or you're gonna go to jail. So when they get that wine, they'll pass it around to finish that bottle so there's no evidence. That happened a lot on the street in town. That does a lot of damage to the person when they drink it all at once. So not many people learned how to be sociable drinkers. They want to drink that wine up because of the law.

When it became legal, it was just like opening a bag of candies to children, you know, they run for it and they went out of control and everybody just sat in bars.

When I came back to the reserve I had been sober for a while. I was talking to this old lady, we were talking about the drinking, and she said, "Remember when we can count people on our hands?"

She meant that there wasn't over ten people that were drinking back then. Today you can't count. Everybody's drinking. You cannot count ten people that are sober today. After the alcohol was opened to the Indians.

GEORGE is a quiet and dignified sixty-nine-year-old Ojibway. A retired teacher, he was interviewed in a seniors' home on the Fort Alexander reserve in southern Manitoba.

I did go into the pubs before they changed the law but I never got served. I was a qualified teacher then. I was teaching regular curriculum at a white school. I was teaching up along Number 6 Highway.

Anyway, I used to stop by Hodgson to have a beer. I tried to. The waiters questioned you, you see. They'd tell me to prove that I am non-treaty. I couldn't prove it, so they'd send me out. They wouldn't serve me. They weren't mad or anything like that. No, they just politely try to find out how your standings are.

Of course I didn't feel so good when they turned me out because I felt like having a drink and I'd have to go without it. I never got really mad 'cause I knew the law required that they had to do that. That's why there wasn't much use getting mad at them for that. I felt it was only right to allow Indian boys to drink government liquor rather than to drink what they used to resort to — perfume, shaving lotion, all that kind of stuff.

FRANK is a fifty-three-year-old Cayuga who grew up in southern Ontario.

At the time when it wasn't possible for Indians to consume alcohol legally, there was a hotel near Hamilton called The Plantation. It was a hotel that would serve native people if you could pass for white. There was this one fella from the reserve, Edwin, who could pass for white, and he was in there having a beer.

The door opens up and in come two fellas from the reserve. Cecil and Roy. But they didn't meet those guidelines. They were dark — Indian written all over them. They went to a table and sat down and the waiter came over and he was quite pleasant about it, he wasn't nasty about it or anything, and he went over and he says, "I'm sorry boys. I can't serve you."

So Cecil and Roy got up and they started to leave the place and they spotted Edwin sitting over at a table there. Cecil went over there and as they passed Edwin's table, they slowed down. He said to Edwin, "When we came in here, I told Roy not to slam the door."

Both Cecil and Roy are gone now but that story still endures because I still hear it every so often when I go home among the older people. Every once in a while you hear somebody say, "Don't slam the door now."

YVONNE *is a short thirty-one-year-old Cree with long black hair. A mother of four children, she grew up on a reserve in northern Alberta.*

I can remember one incident when I was just a kid that happened with the police and my parents before it was legal for treaty Indians to drink. We didn't have electricity at the time and I was about five or six and there was a coal-oil lamp on the table. My parents were drinking, most likely homemade brew, and then I remember my mother got scared 'cause she said, "Cops, cops," in Cree to my father.

They were knocking at the door saying, "Open up. Open up."

My mother, she turned the wick down to where the wick fell into the oil, and it was just pitch dark in the house and I got scared and the police, they knocked the door down. They literally kicked it down on the floor and they searched the whole place. They had these big flashlights. They searched the whole place looking for booze and my parents, they stashed it, and the police they didn't find the booze.

I was just a kid but it's just like it happened yesterday. I remember this 'cause I was terrified.

PAUL, a fifty-nine-year-old teacher, is a Malecite who grew up on the Tobique reserve in New Brunswick.

When they allowed the Indians to vote is when they allowed them to buy liquor, because before then they considered them children — wards, you know — therefore you cannot sell liquor to your children. Even the grand chief around here couldn't buy liquor. With all the stature he had, he had to go to the local bum down the street and ask him to go to the liquor store and buy him a jug of wine or whatever he wanted. He had to lower himself to the street bum to buy liquor for him.

It was humiliation, and consequently the Indians took other means to procure alcohol. They would make their own homebrew. Also, they would drink different things that had alcohol in it, like vanilla extract, lemon extract and canned heat — the same juice that campers use to start

a fire in the woods. I recall my father and grandfather —
they used to put that in a little dirty old rag and they'd
squeeze that rag and the juice would just pour out and
they'd drink that juice.

*MORRIS is a tall and earnest forty-eight-year-old Micmac
with salt-and-pepper hair. He heard about the end of Indian
prohibition in a migrant workers' camp in New Brunswick
when he was fifteen years old.*

I remember it so well. It was in the morning and we were
getting ready to go and pick blueberries. There were some
people from Eel Ground, but most of the people were from
Big Cove. I was the only one from Restigouche there. We
were all Micmacs.

We all stayed in tents and slept on grass. It was a camp.
We were like transient workers, like Mexicans. We walked
to the fields and the white people drove around in cars.
They were the bosses and we were the pickers.

It was a nice day, it was August, that's when the blueberries come out. The owners were parked in front of our
tent. The car doors were open and the radio was on, and
from the news came the announcement that it was offi-
cially passed by Parliament or whatever that it was now
legal to serve liquor to Indian people in Canada.

We all yelled. Actually, it was kind of funny because the
white people didn't understand what was going on. We
had been drinking through bootleggers anyway, even
when I was fifteen, which I regret, having started that
young. But when they announced the fact that we were
able to drink out in the open, it was great news for us
because it meant we didn't have to hide anymore.

There wasn't any celebration. We just kind of yelled and went off to do our business. We didn't do anything different. It was as if to say to the white man, "Hey, look. We're like you guys now."

It didn't really matter. I think most of those people who yelled didn't even drink. It was just the principle of the thing.

JOHN'S STORY

John is a fifty-two-year-old Tlingit who grew up in the Yukon. A dark, hawk-faced man with a quiet, serious demeanour, he speaks in a deep monotone. He was interviewed in his home, a small bungalow near Red Deer, Alberta. He has been sober for nine years.

Back then if we wanted to drink we had to befriend a white man and get him to go down to the bar. I remember getting different people to go down to the bar for me and you only had a certain amount of people who would do it and get you a case of beer.

I got tired of having to pay a person to get beer for me. So the government come up with this idea saying that if you give up your Indian rights, and take the white man's rights, then you're allowed to go and buy liquor. You're allowed to sit in the cocktail lounge or the bars or whatever it might be, and do whatever you want. That sounded great to me, man. I tell you I just went, "Where's the papers? I'll sign them right now."

I got them, signed, and I still got that enfranchisement card, a little blue one. It was your ticket to white society. Or a ticket to alcoholism. A ticket to freedom. The ticket to do whatever the white man did.

I did this in order to buy liquor and to be able to go into beer parlours because that was the "in" thing to do. And I could name a dozen people that have done it.

The funny thing is once you get this little card, it made me feel superior to my own people, my own race. Made me feel better than them because I can go in the bar and they can't. And I was the guy that was getting a commission to go and buy booze for my own people. That's sick. I think back on it now and I'm ashamed of having to do that.

In the last five years they passed another law stating that if I wanted to, I could get back my Indian status. Now I've got another little card that says I'm a 100 percent Indian. (*laughs*) Isn't that crazy?

The people I drank with were much like myself because I wouldn't go in and drink with a doctor. I wouldn't drink with a lawyer. I wouldn't drink with upper crust. It seems like I always drank with people that were at my own level or lower. And then later on, it got to be that I drank with people that were always lower in life than I was because it made me feel superior. It made me feel better than them or not as bad as they are.

When I was nineteen I was arrested for being drunk in a public place up in Whitehorse in the Yukon Territory. I ended up in jail and it was a very scary situation. I'd never been in jail in my life. I didn't know what it was like to sleep on a hard concrete floor that was cold. I didn't know what it was like to have to go to the bathroom in the presence of fifteen other people who were crammed into a little cell about nine-by-twelve. The following morning when I went to court, I was very scared. I didn't have money for my fine, which was fifteen dollars. I didn't know how I was going to pay and I worried about this for quite some time. They gave me two weeks to pay.

I remember going down to the newspaper because at that time they used to print the stories about the different people that ended up in the drunk tank. My friends would read these things and they would laugh about different people going to jail. So I didn't want to "make the papers" as we used to say. I went down with the intention of trying to bribe the newspaper editor, to pay him twenty dollars to keep my name out of the paper. At that time twenty dollars was quite a substantial amount of money. Fifteen dollars was a big pile of money. I didn't want to be singled out. I didn't want to be made a fool of. I didn't want people laughing at me. I didn't want people to know I was in jail for being drunk in a public place. The editor just said, "If it goes in, it goes in. I can't control that." But I think he felt sorry for me because I didn't see it in the paper the next day. I was very thankful for that. I didn't bribe him.

I just about killed my brother one time. I felt like he deserved it. He went to bed with one of the best girlfriends I ever had. I found her in bed with him and I took a beer bottle, snapped the end of it off and took it to his throat. I thought I killed him. I was drunk at the time and I left. If I'd a known that he hadn't died at that time, I probably would have killed him because I was hurt very much and very deeply. Because with all the women in the world, why did he have to pick on mine?

I don't know whether it was because he did that to me or what, but I found in later years I was doing the same thing to other people. If I saw a man with a woman and they were happy, I had to do something to break it up. Seems weird. It took me a long time for me to forgive my brother for that. Now we can talk to each other but we don't talk about it.

I lost two of my brothers to alcohol. I lost a nephew. I

lost my brother-in-law. They all drank themselves to death. It cost me one marriage, alcoholism cost me that. And it's a heavy price to pay. It's a price I never want to pay again. The effect of alcohol on my community is also very expensive because in the last fifteen years the place where I was born and raised, nearly all those old boys have died, both men and women, and I'd say about 85 percent of them have died of alcoholism.

When did I make the decision to stay sober? It happened on July 29, 1981, at approximately 11:30 in the morning, after I drank a bottle of vodka. I was too drunk to go to work. I was too drunk to walk. I was too drunk to think and too drunk to talk. I was in a hopeless situation where I thought of taking my own life. I was at a point in my life where I think I was the lowest possible that I could possibly get. I was hopelessly lost in alcohol. I didn't give a damn about anybody or anything. It was either blow my brains out or find help.

I was scared to look for help because I didn't know where to look and I didn't know who to turn to. I knew there was a God somewhere. I got down on my hands and knees by my bed, I remember that, and I prayed to God.

I said, "God, if You're there, please help me."

From that day to now, I never had to have another drink. So he's heard my prayer.

Later I went to a dry-out centre in Calgary. They showed me a film on alcohol and what it did to my brain cells every time I drank. It's up in the thousands of brain cells that died each time I got drunk. And that's what scared me into becoming really sincere about stopping. That film scared me so much because I had been drinking so long. I drank for twenty-some years and I mean real hard drinking, lots of it. I drank for two years prior to sobering up, without stopping. I realized that if I kept up this way I wouldn't have any brain left. I realized that I really did a lot of damage to my brain and I'm lucky to be where I am today.

I mean, someone can tell you, "John, if you don't quit drinking, you're going to die." Many, many people have told me that, my doctor included. It wasn't until I saw it on film, on a screen. I think it's something people should see.

I ended up going to my first AA meeting on August 1, 1981, in Red Deer. I was scared because I was the only Indian in the meeting. Yet these people, there were about forty people in the meeting, they stuck their hand out. They didn't look at my colour or they didn't look at who I was or what I was. They welcomed me and after the meeting they said, "Please come back because we need you."

No one in my whole life had ever said that to me. No one had ever said, "John, we want you to come back." That kept me going back until this day.

AA has given me a chance to live. At one time I didn't know the meaning of the word "live." I knew what it was like to exist. I know what it is like to live from day to day wondering what the hell life is all about, or if life had reason, or if there was reason to live. Because I didn't know.

The best thing I like about sobriety today is the freedom. The freedom from fear. The freedom from wondering what the hell I did yesterday. And the freedom from booze. The freedom to live life as I see it today.

My life today has turned around completely from what it was before. Today I find that I love my fellow man. Today I find that I can talk to different women without wondering what it would be like to make love to them. Today I can talk to different men without wondering what I could get out of them.

I find that I can look someone in the eye, in the face, and tell them that I care for them. And I find that people care for me. And I find that life is worth living. I found a new way of living through the AA program and I found that it didn't matter who the hell you were, where you came from, what you did, whether you were a doctor or a lawyer, merchant or a judge. It didn't matter whether you're Indian or white or black or Chinese or Japanese or whatever you are — the help is there for everybody. Today I know there's hope in life. When I first came into this program, there was no hope. I thought I had to die an alcoholic. I am going to die an alcoholic, but if I stay in this program, I'm going to die a sober alcoholic. And for anyone who's looking for a place to sober up, I recommend strongly that they go to AA because it saved my life.

3

THE FIRST TIME

"That was the best thing I ever tasted. It just gave me a sensation I'll never forget . . . I knew that alcohol was something special. I knew I was going to pursue alcohol as much as I could in the future."

The first drinking experience for most non-native Canadians is in many ways quite different from the first drinking experience of native people. Many Canadians probably have their first taste of alcohol at the family dinner table when they have been invited to sip from a glass of beer or a watered-down glass of wine. The first drink of many native people, however, is usually nowhere nearly as genteel. It is usually a hurried and secretive affair that doesn't end until the first-time drinker passes out. These first-time drinkers — children usually — pass out because they drink large quantities of homebrew, moonshine, hard liquor or fortified wine.

Given the combination of these furtive and dangerous circumstances, the first drinking experience of many native people is often a horrible event.

❧

LAZARUS is the husky, smiling seventy-four-year-old elder from the Stoney reserve in southern Alberta who said in Chapter 1 that the word for alcohol in his language meant "crazywater." He is a retired rancher.

In 1936, my brother Paul was staying here with his wife. I was about twenty. We were doing the trapping for some squirrels, weasels, mink, coyotes and so on. Paul, another buddy of mine by the name of Louis and his dad — four of us — were taking our fur to Bragg Creek. We went over there, sold the pelts, and this fur-buyer was also a bootlegger. My brother Paul bought a jug of wine. So on the way back home, he stopped and he gave my buddy a drink. He took a good drink. He must have drinken before, my buddy.

My brother gave me the jug of wine. I took it. It was cold and I was shivering. So I took a good drink and, oh, it sounds funny, pretty soon like my head is gonna burst. My eyes open like this (*his eyes widen*) and then my fingers begin to tickle and something funny happened. "Hey, it seems like I'm gonna get sick, give me some more."

So I took another. My buddy's father, he wasn't drinking, so between three of us we finished one gallon of wine. Of course we were pretty drunk. But we can find our way back. We were on horseback. I didn't get passed out but I was drunk by the time I got back. That's the first time I started to drink.

Later on, some boys, my buddies, came along. "Hey, we got a bottle here, would you like to take a drink?"

"Yeah." I took a drink.

"Hey, take another snort." So that's how it got worse and worse, and finally I can't stop drinking even though I wanted to, I couldn't do it.

⚭

GERALDINE *is a thirty-six-year-old Tlingit. She grew up in a small village in the Yukon.*

I was about twelve years old and I was with my cousin Darlene who was a year younger than me. We stole about eight bottles of wine off her dad and we both got very, very drunk.

I was living with my grandparents and when we got home my grandfather at first didn't really realize what was going on. But when he saw that I was having trouble undoing my coat he realized I was drunk and he sent me to bed.

We lived in this old house. My bed was upstairs and if I sat up too quick I'd bump my head on the ceiling. So anyway, I was in bed and I was laying there and I started getting really sick. I was puking and the puke was going up and hitting the ceiling and coming back down all over me.

Next day everything was so stink and my hair was all matted with this puke and I had to run outside and get sick all over again. I really got a lot of shit. My grandmother was just hollering and screaming at me and everything.

She made me scrub all my blankets. We didn't have running water or anything then. We had to haul water from the river and heat it up, put it in the tub and scrub all our clothes by hand. So that day was spent washing my hair and then scrubbing the blankets all day and the sheets and my clothes and everything.

I was really sick and my friends were upset because they thought I got them in trouble. It was a lot of to-do about it.

I never, ever talk about that incident and when people would bring it up later on I would tell them to shut up.

LONE EAGLE is a thirty-year-old Ojibway. Wide-eyed, fast-talking and street-wise, he grew up in southern Manitoba.

I remember drinking around the age of eight years old. My parents wanted to get me drunk and see what I was like. There was a party, a lot of people around, all the relatives.

It was crazy. I was eight years old and I was drinking. They put sunglasses on me and gave me a bottle of beer to carry around. That's how it started. I went along with it and didn't know what the hell I was doing. It was a big joke to them. Everybody was laughing. I didn't know what was going on myself. I thought it was okay. I felt good 'cause I was feeling accepted and part of whatever was happening.

The next time I remember getting drunk was when I was around ten years old. I stole a bottle of whiskey from my friend's father and I got really really drunk. I passed out in the arena on my reserve. I vomited on myself that night. I stayed in the arena all by myself all night. They come and got me early the next morning. My brother and my sister found out I was there. They carried me out and I was sick. I was still drunk. They put me on top of the car, facing down on the top of the car, not the hood or the trunk, but on top of the car, and they were holding my hands on each side of the window. (*laughs*) They didn't want me in the car 'cause I was sick on myself.

It was more funny to my parents than actually stealing the bottle of whiskey. The fact that I was so drunk was funnier than the fact that I stole the whiskey. My parents just accepted that.

GARY'S STORY

Gary is a tall and thin, fast-talking thirty-six-year-old Cree. He is studying social work at university and was interviewed in a split-level house in a Calgary suburb. He has been sober for four years.

The first time I took a drink I was fourteen years old. I was in a foster home, my brother was celebrating his eighteenth birthday. He got a gift from his mum and dad which was a bottle of cognac. A mickey. So my brother decided to share it. We lived on a farm and we went outside. He took a drink and he passed it to me and I took a drink and then he put the cork on the bottle and was gonna go away. So I kinda nudged him and asked him for another drink. So he takes another drink and I take another drink and we ended up having about three drinks. But he just corked it up and put it away and I couldn't get my mind off that bottle. Like I couldn't understand why he didn't want to finish drinking that bottle. I wanted to finish it.

So, like, that was my first experience. I never really got drunk or anything, but I'll never forget that, you know, questioning why he wouldn't finish that bottle. I wanted to finish it because I liked it so much. Like, to me, that was the best thing I ever tasted. It just gave me a sensation I'll never forget. A head-to-toe warm feeling. Kind of an uplifting feeling. When I felt that sensation, that's when I knew that alcohol was something special. I knew I was going to pursue alcohol as much as I could in the future.

I lived in a rural farm community with Ukrainian

people. Like there was me and a friend of mine and we were the only two Indian people in the community. When I started drinking I was in grade eleven. I was really a shy person. I was also one of two native people in the community and I didn't fit in and alcohol was something that I could latch onto. I couldn't do anything else. Like I wasn't any good at sports. I wasn't good with women. But one thing I could do was drink and that's what I did. Like right from the very beginning.

I could outdrink people. I could drink whiskey straight. I was the drinker. Like I was always the one who was carried home from the party or I might have barfed all over the place. Like, you know, I always got plastered. That was in high school. I got carried home lots of times from parties and it was a big laugh, you know, and I enjoyed that attention. Like I enjoyed people talking about the fun that we had and I didn't care if I passed out or got carried home. That was great. Like people were finally talking about me. So like it was good.

I was a pig when I drank. I always had that problem even to the last day of drinking. I always used to choke on my beer or I'd take a drink and I'd cough 'cause I drank too fast. Like I could take a shot of whiskey in just one gulp. Three gulps and a beer's gone. I always drank really fast.

I started going to the bar when I was seventeen and I went to the bar every day. I never missed. Plus the liquor stores. And I always had booze in my car. I never missed a day of drinking. I started when I was seventeen and drank till I was thirty-two. My whole life revolved around drinking. Like I never had a plan in life. I never had a goal or anything. All I knew was that I enjoyed drinking.

I always got to know the waiters. And they always knew me on a first-name basis. If I didn't have money, they would buy me drinks. I could go into bars, sit down, call the waiter over and say, you know, "I don't have any money today."

And he'd buy me beer for the whole day. And I'd come back in two days when I had the money and pay him back, give him a tip, square everything up. I could cash cheques in any bar. Like I used to be a regular customer so I could always cash my paycheques there. And if I didn't have money I could cash a personal cheque there. I liked that. I really felt that I was somebody, like I was a valuable customer. It was sort of like an honour, you know. I'd walk in the bar, sit down. You know, people waving for the waiter, right? Well, I didn't do that. As soon as I sit down, my two beers are dropped on the table. So I always liked that rapport that I had established. It used to feel good.

But I never really thought of it as controlling my life. It's just that I couldn't go anywhere or wouldn't do anything unless it had something to do with drinking. And if I had to go somewhere and, say, visit somebody that didn't drink, well I'd drink before and then it would be a very short visit. Just in and out. Eventually I didn't visit anybody that didn't drink.

Where I was raised there was no drugs at all. But it didn't take long before people started offering me grass. My initial reaction to smoking pot was, I lost control. Like I used to drink so much that the combination of drugs and alcohol used to just knock me flat on my ass. I'd start falling down and lose my balance when I combined drugs with alcohol. I would drive and I'd hit the ditch all the time. So the only time I could smoke pot was if I hadn't had a lot of alcohol in me that day.

I wasn't afraid to drink too much. I had done so much drinking I knew I could function even if I was in a blackout. Like I knew I wouldn't do anything stupid. I still had some sense of control when I was in a blackout. But if I had mixed drugs, then I would lose it. It was just a little bit more dangerous.

In 1978 was when I first began to realize that I was having some problems. By then I had had three impaired driving charges. People were starting to tell me, "Gary, you should do something about your drinking."

I was starting to get the shakes. I couldn't control my hands. I was a restaurant manager and you're supposed to socialize with your customers and I'd get these uncontrollable fits of shaking. It happened at the most inopportune times. Like I remember one time my foster mum and dad came to visit me in Vancouver. And at the time I had been on an extraordinarily long binge. Like I was just sick. And my mum and dad surprised me and all of a sudden I started shaking and I couldn't stop. And like I couldn't smoke a cigarette. I just remember putting my hands on the table and just holding on and sitting there. And like wanting them to leave 'cause I almost lost control of my body movements.

And that was beginning to happen quite frequently. Sometimes I'd be standing and all of a sudden I'd start getting nauseated and lose my balance and I'd have to grab onto a table or a wall or something. Plus I was getting some enormous hangovers.

Like it would take me hours to get going in the morning. I'd get up and I'd spend an hour in the washroom just trying to get myself together. Have a shower. Sometimes I'd have two, three showers in a row. I'd get to work and soon as I'd get to work, I'd go to the washroom and I'd spend about a half-hour in there. I'd wash myself. Wash my face. Barf some more. I'd get all pale and I'd sit there and wait till the colour came back in my face. And then I'd walk right through the restaurant, straight into the office and then I'd close the door and I'd sit there maybe for another half-hour. So like the whole process would take about two hours just to get goin' in the morning.

And then in 1978 an employee of mine, she was a waitress, she said that she wanted to talk to me. Like I was the manager, eh, and I thought she was going to complain about her job or something, right?

So we sat down and I said, "What do you want to talk about?"

And she said, "It's about your drinking. I know that you drink a lot and I think that if you don't quit drinking you're gonna get yourself into some trouble."

And I, of course, was very defensive. I cut her off really abruptly and told her that it was none of her business. I was the manager and she was a waitress and if she valued her job she wouldn't go around criticizing the manager.

She was older than me, like, she was a family person. She was just trying to direct me to Alcoholics Anonymous 'cause she had a member of her family in the program. But I didn't wait around and listen for her whole speech. I just cut her off.

I haven't seen this woman since, but she planted a seed in my head. I never forget that. Like I was really hurt and offended and you know it was a real attack against me. What happened was I ended up quitting my job very shortly after that. I quit and I moved.

That was my way of dealing with problems. I'd pack up and move. I'd pack everything in the station wagon, grab my kids and I take off. I had no idea where I was going or what I was gonna do. But I was gone and I'd leave my problems behind. That's what I did. In my adult life I did that over twenty times. Packed up and moved and just said, "Forget it. Que sera sera." I'd get an unlisted phone number and nobody'd ever know where I was or where I went.

The way I sobered up was this. I phoned Alcoholics Anonymous on June 12, 1987, here in Calgary. I was probably days away from giving my kids up to welfare 'cause I no longer could look after my kids. That's when I knew I was an alcoholic.

I was broke. I filed for bankruptcy. Like I used to own a home. I used to have two cars and a three-bedroom house with everything in it. I had a colour television, stereo, fridge, stove, washer, dryer, microwave. We owned all that stuff. I was making $30,000 a year and finally I lost my job. I was broke. I couldn't look after my kids anymore. I just knew that I had to quit drinking.

When I finished my last beer at three o'clock in the morning, I phoned AA and they sent somebody over. I was ready. So that's basically how I sobered up and I stayed sober through the help of AA. But the first year, like it was long, it was hard and it was tough. More than once I thought, "How am I going to live the rest of my life without drinking?" You know? "I might as well be dead because there's nothing left in life if I can't have a drink. This is ridiculous."

But that's where the AA program came in. It really helped me to quit drinking. And instilled some things in me to understand about the disease of alcoholism and why I couldn't drink.

I also had this Indian-ness problem. I didn't know my birth family and I also didn't know Indian people. I associated with Indian people but only in a drinking context. Like I'd go to a bar and I'd search out an Indian person and I'd go and buy him a beer and I'd sit with him and talk and drink. I'd go to Indian parties. I drank with them on skid row. I'd drink on the reserve with them. I wanted to be an Indian but I wasn't really an Indian, I didn't know anything about myself.

So after a year of sobriety I went to a native treatment centre — Poundmaker's Lodge — and there I learned a lot about Indian people and Indian culture. Like some really profound things happened to me there. Everybody had the same story. We were all uprooted from our families. None of us knew anything about Indian people. Like here we are, we were all adults and they were teaching us about Indian people. So all of a sudden it dawned on me that I wasn't alone out there anymore. I was suffering the same disease and I had the same symptoms and this was really profound because there was native people from all across Canada there.

That's when I realized that I had to build some new relationships in my life. Like I used to subscribe to middle-class values 'cause I was raised by white, middle-class people. I used to subscribe to those values and I used to be very materialistic. I used to suffer a lot of anxiety over money and prestige and a job and status and, like, I threw all that stuff out the window. I decided the most important thing in my life was to be Indian and to get to know Indian people.

Like one of the most profound things that happened to me there was I realized Indian people were human beings just like everybody else. Somehow I had this idea that Indian people were less than human beings. They were, you know, just drunks. They had no feelings, they didn't cry. They had no motivation, no goals, ambitions, dreams or anything. They had nothing. They were just faceless, nameless people.

I had never seen an Indian cry before I went to the treatment centre and to see them crying and to see them hurting was when I realized that they were very special people and I wanted to get to know them. I learned at Poundmaker's it's okay to be an Indian.

Like those things happening to me made me want to get in touch with my historical roots, to get to know Indian people. I did that through my birth family. I got to know them really well since I sobered up, and I formed some very close relationships. I found that there's a lot of alcoholism in my family. My mother's an alcoholic and she had other children that she had given up because of her alcohol problem. I don't know who my father is. My grandfather was an alcoholic and so was my great-grandfather. And there's been a lot of tragedies in my family.

But that's been the history of Indian people. There's been a lot of displacement. They've been displaced from their land and their culture and from their history and from their language. And that's the history of my family. The history of what happened to the Indian people is what happened to my family. They were displaced from the land and their way of life and that's what happened to me. The same thing. I was displaced from Indian people, and alcohol helped me forget that displacement. It just blotted everything out of my mind. Like I didn't belong in this world and so I drank.

Today it's not like that. Like I really feel good about my family and I always feel really comfortable with Indian people. Like I have a very rich history as far as my family goes. I feel very proud about my family. I see the elders and I'm learning about the culture and I socialize and I have a circle of native friends. I was able to sort a lot of things out and feel good about who I am.

Like I remember being in Poundmaker's and my counsellor asked me if I had ever looked myself in the mirror and told myself that I loved Gary, that Gary was a good person. I'd never done that. I could never look at myself in the mirror. As a matter of fact I could never look people in the eye. When I talked to people I always looked on the ground. I could never look at the same level as people. I was always below them and I felt very inferior. That day in Poundmaker's I was in my room and I looked in the mirror and it was very hard for me to say it but I said it. And from then on I still have to discipline myself to hold myself up and be proud of who I am, proud of my ancestry, proud of my family and proud of Indian people. I guess that was about the biggest thing that happened to me there. I got my self-esteem back and an identity.

That's how confused I was. I was told for so long by my foster family that I wasn't an Indian. Nobody ever told me that I *was* an Indian. And so, you know like I was really lost. Like I was thirty-three years old and I didn't have an identity. I didn't know who I was and where I belonged. Poundmaker's gave me an identity. They gave me a base and a foundation to work on and I've been growing from there.

Religion and spirituality, that's another thing that Poundmaker's gave me. They gave me some stuff I could take home and practise in my everyday life — Indian spirituality.

I was raised in a Roman Catholic convent for five years. I turned away from believing in anything. I didn't believe there was a God. I had lost all faith in religion, but native spirituality was something I trusted. They gave it to me and told me that I could use it and I did.

I started going to sweats [sweat lodges]. I started burning sweetgrass. And I started believing. I like the concept of Mother Earth and of Nature and of all things being equal. And everybody living in harmony and in unison and one person not being any better than the other one. I like the idea of decisions by consensus and getting to know my family and loving my family. Seeing the good in people. Not being critical.

I think spiritually now. As I go through the day I try to be a spiritual person. I don't make decisions based on self-ishness and self-will. It's a bit of AA philosophy and Indian philosophy.

Even my thoughts have changed. I have goals. Like I never had goals before. I have a vision of what I want to do and how I want to live out my life. Like I never had any of that before. I'm even looking forward to being an old person. So it's been very settling.

My life's taken a whole new direction and meaning. In 1986 I filed for bankruptcy. I didn't have a cent to my name. I lost all my credit cards. My daughters and I were living in a sleeping room. We had one bed and everything we owned was in that room. Then we moved to a three-bedroom apartment, but we had no furniture.

Not only has my financial situation changed, my philosophy has changed about materialism and stuff like that. All of a sudden I didn't need the things that I had before. They weren't important. If I need something now, I save the money up for it and I just pay cash. Like that was probably the best thing that ever happened to me, going bankrupt, 'cause I was able to start fresh again.

Today, my wife and I don't owe any money. We don't own a hell of a lot. We rent the house and we got a couple a ten-year-old cars, but we don't owe a cent to anybody. We have financial freedom. I'm not constrained by the banks and the mortgage companies and the credit institutions and I don't plan to be. I don't plan on getting a mortgage. I don't plan on buying a car or anything on a loan. If I don't have the money, I'm not going to buy it. That's the way I plan to live for the rest of my life. If we wanted to move, we could. We'd just have a little garage sale and get rid of our stuff here and take off.

We as a family have a lot of problems. But one thing that we do today that I'd never do before is get help. Like I strongly believe in counselling, working out issues, resolving resentments and fears and angers. You know, forming intimate relationships, not the surface-level type. Like really talking about your feelings and talking about things that really matter. Like the real human-level conversation about "How are you today?" and "How are you feeling?" Like "What's on your mind? What's bothering you?" And, you know, just getting things out on the table. That's what we're working towards. We haven't achieved that yet because we have a lot of blocks and unresolved issues, but we're working towards it.

We're heavily involved in self-help programs for alcoholics, families of alcoholics, children of alcoholics, you know, plus counselling, family counselling and one-on-one counselling. It's necessary for us to function and to stay together as a family. Because I know that if I don't make it in this relationship, I won't make it in the next relationship. And if my children don't resolve these issues now they will have the same problems that I had.

It's a family disease. It's a cyclical thing and unless we break the cycle right now, we will not enjoy any freedom or happiness until we sort this stuff all out. We want very much to have a good relationship, but it's very difficult for us. We keep getting dragged down by things that have happened to us as children. We have to recognize that it's not because of who we are, it's because of the way we were brought up. But we're gonna break that. We're gonna beat it and we're gonna have a good relationship. In spite of all that stuff.

One of the reasons I'm going into social work is because I don't ever want a native foster child to go through what I had to go through. I lived in some very abusive foster homes. I was physically, emotionally and sexually abused in more than one foster home. I was one of the luckier ones. I really didn't get harmed that bad. But like I want to make sure that that doesn't happen again. Native people should be raised in native foster homes. Native people shouldn't be separated from their siblings and they shouldn't be separated from their language. And if at all possible, they should be given some Indian-ness some- how, somewhere along the line and not just be totally cut off.

It's very easy to find sober native people. The unfortu- nate thing is that a drunken Indian lying down on skid row is very visible in the city. Nobody talks about the thou- sands of Indians in the communities. There's thousands of sober people out there. Those are my role models. I get my strength from going out there and seeing them in their everyday life, getting along without alcohol.

There's a renewal. That's a word I like. There's a renew- al in the Indian community and I'm glad that I'm a part of it.

4

BINGEING, BOOTLEGGING AND RACISM

"Yeah, I do have a drinking problem. I like the taste of booze and when I start, I can't stop."

Binge drinkers do not drink every day and they often go for extended periods without touching a drop. But when they start on a binge, the intense, compulsive drinking can continue non-stop for days, weeks and months. At its worst, binge drinking is a suicidal routine — one binge quickly followed by another and another — that ends in death.

Compared to non-native drinkers, Indian drinkers are twice as likely to be binge drinkers, according to recent studies. The roots of Indian binge drinking may go back thousands of years — to a time when Indian people lived a cyclical existence, dependent on the harvest of fish, game and plantlife. Then, the harvest season was a time of feasting and celebration. The feast was a central element of Indian life and it was against this historical and cultural backdrop that Indian people came into contact with alcohol. If their traditions were not reason enough, Indian people soon evolved a binge drinking culture under the influence of the first Europeans. Rowdy soldiers and adventurers set a hard-drinking example while greedy whiskey sellers and fur-traders actively promoted binge drinking.

Whatever its roots, binge drinking is now a prominent feature of native drinking and is quite distinct from the "social" drinking pattern of non-native people.

Native drinking is different from non-native drinking in other ways as well. For example, native people rely on bootleggers and homemade alcohol far more than non-native people do. And if drinking and its effects weren't bad enough, native people also have to contend with racism as a regular and infuriating element of their drinking environment.

ANGELA is a Cree from northern Manitoba. She is forty years old but looks much older. Her front teeth are missing and the bridge of her nose was smashed flat into her face some time ago. She was interviewed in a native treatment centre. It was her sixth time in treatment.

I wasn't a social drinker, that's for sure. I drank heavy. I drank every day. I drank without eating. I drank Lysol, Listerine, rubbing alcohol, after-shave. You name it, I drank them all. I seen people drinking them. They were feeling good, so I figured I might as well drink them, eh?

You mix Lysol with water, lukewarm water. You mix it in a big bottle. That tall part, whatchyoucallit, the foam, that has to settle down first, then you drink it. Rubbie (rubbing alcohol) and after-shave you just put cold water. Listerine is 22 percent alcohol, you drink it straight.

Lysol used to make me sick right around here. (*rubs her stomach*) Make me sick. I just keep wishing I would die. But I guess I wasn't ready to go. (*laughs*) I wanted to kill myself lots of times. I thought nobody liked me.

A lot of times I end up in the hospital after getting beaten up. Lots of times I'd have blackouts and end up in jail. If I didn't have money, I'd go steal. I got arrested one time for stealing Listerine. I drank anything I got my hands on.

REBECCA *is a short, fashionably dressed Blood in her early twenties. She was interviewed in a native treatment centre at the end of a four-week program.*

I have yet to meet an Indian social drinker. Some say they're social drinkers and they can go out for a couple of beer, but at one occasion or another you see them drunk. They say they're social drinkers but they still get drunk.

I have white friends who are social drinkers who *every time* they say, "Let's go out for a drink," they'll only have one or two, you know, every time. I've never seen them drunk. So I don't think drinking is for Indians.

LONE EAGLE *is a short, stocky thirty-year-old Manitoba Ojibway with an explosive laugh. He was interviewed after four weeks in a native treatment centre.*

I usually drink with lower-class, down-and-out kind of people, people that don't really care to dress up, look a little dirty, basically people that don't care much about themselves. I feel comfortable drinking with these people, I don't know why.

I don't drink with high-class people because they're so cheap. (*laughs*) They'd have a fat bank account and they'd get drunk, but that's it. They'd stop at a one-drunk session. I can't drink like that. I'm an alcoholic.

Native people go all out. I'm not afraid to spend $300 a night, whereas the white person will be conservative and not want to spend that much money. They're cheap and I just don't feel comfortable with them. I want to find somebody that's gonna devote all of their time and all of their money in a drinking session with me (*laughs*) and there is people like that. There is. Believe it or not, there is.

I'll spend everything I got on a drinking session. If I got $500 and I decide to drink, I'll spend it all. I won't quit drinking till it's all gone. No matter how long it takes. Just keep drinking. Just don't stop. Bad habit but that's what I do. It's nothing for me to buy twenty cases of beer. I can't drink twenty cases myself, but I buy that 'cause I know there's gonna be other people there and we share.

When we go to parties, I'll bring four twenty-fours, where white people will bring just a twelve. And then they drink ours after theirs is gone. That's the difference between white people and native people in my experience.

ALFRED *is a quiet, shy thirty-seven-year-old Cree from a tiny, isolated community in northern Manitoba.*

Bootleggers used to make me mad. They wouldn't let me charge up drinks. There was one bootlegger in Moose Lake. I went and bought bootleg stuff, a twenty-four case of beer for fifty bucks.

I was half-drunk and I had no money so I tried this just to get a drink. A two-dollar bill is red, so is a fifty-dollar bill. So I wrote on one side, "$50." I fold it up (*laughs*) and gave it to her. I just thought I'd try it.

I turned that two-dollar bill to a fifty. She didn't look at it, just grabbed it and put it in her pocket and (*laughs*) gave me the twenty-four. She was in a hurry, I guess. She didn't check that money and it worked.

She couldn't tell the cops after. (*laughs*) She would have told on herself. But she was after me for a long time. She was an old lady, she's dead now. She started arguing with me every time I seen her till the day she died. (*laughs*) I never forget that.

WILMA *is a fifty-two-year-old Mohawk grandmother who grew up on the Six Nations Grand River Territory in southern Ontario.*

I saw all the drunks at their worst, when they came to buy booze from my ma, who by the way was a bootlegger during the Depression years so she could support her kids. So I've got mixed feelings about bootlegging because I might have starved to death if my mother had not sold enough booze to buy food to feed me.

My mother was a bootlegger when alcohol was prohibited on the reserve. And as a kid during those times I can remember the RCMP coming to raid our place and we used to watch them go through the whole house looking for the hiding places and we knew where the hiding places were but we knew better than to open our mouth.

My grandfather was my mother's role model. Her father. He was a bootlegger too and he made homebrew and he drank his own stuff and eventually he hemorrhaged and passed out and fell face forward in his own pool of blood and that was how he died.

DOMINICK *is a wiry, grizzled fifty-three-year-old Cree. He was interviewed on the streets of Thompson, Manitoba, and was obviously drunk.*

In the pubs here, any pub, eh? When Indian go in the pub, if there's no room, Indians go out first and they let white guys go and have a beer. You know what I mean?

If I go in a bar, and Indian talk rough, you go out. But white guys when they talking rough in the bar, they don't bother them. They just laugh at them. They figure they're fun. But an Indian when they start talking about the same goddam thing as the white man — out. Bouncer throw you out.

What's a difference? A white man and an Indian. What's the difference?

KATHY *is a fair-skinned forty-five-year-old Cree with wide brown eyes. She is smartly dressed in a red sweater and a black leather skirt. She grew up in British Columbia and worked as a bartender almost all of her adult life. She has been sober for five years and is now a real estate agent. She was interviewed in a Vancouver hotel room.*

I went to work for a very short time up in Kamloops. I got a job in the beer parlour there. This was probably twenty years ago. It was mostly construction workers that came in. I guess I'd been working for four or five days and a group of Indians came in and the bartender says to me, "Don't serve them."

This was a family, I can still remember them. There was a big, large mother, she was really heavy, and the old man and a daughter. They weren't drunk, and I said, "Why not?"

And he said, "We don't serve Indian people in here."

So I said, "Well how do you feel about *them* people working in here?"

He says, "Oh, fuck no." (*laughs*) So I threw my tray on him and climbed over the bar and tried to kill him. The Indians came and rescued me and off we went to the Indian bar across the street. I quit on the spot. I had to. I was trying to kill him.

That's pretty well how people who work in bars feel about Indians. Like the Legion, they don't want Indians in there. I know it. I went to work at the Legion on Hastings Street. I would be working on the floor and it was expected that if an Indian couple came in and got into a fight, they'd say, "Well, you knew that was coming. What did you serve them for?"

This might have happened three times in the seven years I worked there, that an Indian party would erupt into a fight, but it was always taken for granted that it would happen. I would be working on the floor and everyone would say, "*Oh, God*, there's a drunken Indian. How we gonna get him out of here?" You know? Meanwhile, all the white people in there are drunk.

They're inherently prejudiced towards Indians. People talk like this around me and in front of me because they think I'm white or it doesn't occur to them.

There's definitely an attitude. When you *first* come in and you're an Indian, they think you shouldn't be there.

They don't care if Indians were in the service. They don't want Indian veterans in there.

ITGAQ'S STORY

Itgaq is a forty-three-year-old Yupik broadcaster in Alaska. He has an angular face, with high cheekbones and a pointed chin. He talks with his granny glasses off and his eyes squeezed shut. He calls himself a binge drinker and says he hasn't had a drink in the past two weeks. He was interviewed in a cramped studio in the village radio station.

When I first started drinking, the thing that impressed me the most was that it made me feel more energetic, a little stronger. It seemed like I could do more work. If I had a few drinks, by golly, I could go out and work in the garden or clean the yard or do stuff like that. It made me want to work, work, work. When I was young, I could drink and work or go out dancing and have fun and not get drunk.

But nowadays, I get a jug and I'll just sit there and drink until I get so drunk I don't know what I'm doing anymore. I *can't* stop. I have *one* drink and then when it's finished, I have to pour another one. I continue to drink until I *pass out*. There has to be *no more booze* in the house for me to quit drinking. Usually I only drink on weekends because I don't want to jeopardize my job. But then sometimes it'll go over the weekend to Friday. I miss that whole week on the drunk. That's what usually happens to me.

I do my drinking at home alone. Usually I invite a friend of mine, a neighbour, over and he'll come in and drink with me. I don't usually like to drink alone. If I do, then I've got my TV set full blast. At least I'm not just sitting there watching the jug.

If I really want to get drunk, I'll buy two or three jugs of booze. This is a dry town so I gotta buy them from a bootlegger. They're only seven bucks or something in Anchorage right now, but here they're fifty bucks. So sometimes I can spend a hundred and fifty bucks in a day on three fifths of booze. And because the booze costs so damn much, it seems like if a person buys a fifth, he has to drink it alone 'cause it costs so doggone much (*laughs*) to share with somebody else. Heck, maybe that's how come I like to drink alone. Maybe if they had a liquor store and the price went down, heck, then I'd be drinking with everybody else.

When I'm drinking I don't give a damn about my work, about how I live or whether I eat or not. I just have an I-don't-care attitude about *myself*. But I care about other people when I'm drinking. I care about how other people see me. That's why I don't go out when I'm drinking. I sit at home and I get drunk and I pass out on the floor. I never walk around downtown 'cause if I walk around town drunk, then they say, "*Oh, he's a drunk.*" I don't want them to think of me as a drunk.

I've tried to quit drinking and sometimes I can quit for months on end. I just say, "The heck with it." I don't want it, I just don't want to taste it or smell it or be around people who drink. But then I get angry at some-body or some situation and that gets me started again. I don't know how many times I've tried to quit drink-ing — probably around five, six times. But there'd be some kind of a happy occasion and I'd have a drink here, next time a little bit more and I'd be back into drinking again.

A friend of mine talked me into going to a detox centre in Anchorage. I told him I've got this really beautiful dog I don't want nothing to happen to it, middle of the winter and stuff like that. The dog was home alone and I don't want nothing to happen to that dog.

I went to a treatment centre for a whole month. I had no problems except their program was bringing stuff out that was inside of me that I didn't know was there, and all that stuff that I was bringing out kind of made me *angry* because it was coming out into the open and I was telling somebody else that I was having problems. I felt obligated to talk about my problems there because that was part of the program. If you wanted to get out of there, you better say what they want to hear and write what they want to read, so I did all that.

There was this one step at the end, I forgot if it was the fifth step or sixth step, before you could leave, you had to write down something. So I just *faked it all* and they believed me and I got out that same weekend. Other guys didn't make it but I convinced them that I was cured. (*laughs*) I must be a good liar. In my farewell talk to them, I was talking to them about, "Oh, it's a beautiful life and all." They believed me. (*laughs*) I really wanted to get out and I had to convince them, so I made it real *good*, I mean really convincing.

When I left there I went straight to the Alaska Federation of Natives, their final day banquet or something. I saw a whole bunch of friends from my home town, so I sat with them. Pretty soon this waitress came along and everybody ordered beer. I had just gotten out of the hospital that same day, just graduated or whatever, and I said, "Gee, I wonder if I should?"

And they said, "Sure, just one beer won't hurt you." (*laughs*) So I had one beer *and another and another. I really had a lot of fun.*

But when I came home my dog was dead. I had told my neighbours to take care of it and they didn't. I was so damn mad over that dog that I never forgave that guy who talked me into trying to stop drinking, so I just started drinking again.

In general, I think native people drink too much because they feel inadequate in that they are no longer a provider for their family. Years and years ago they used to go out and *hunt*, they used to go out and *trap*, they used to go out and *fish* for the family.

Nowadays there are so many rules and regulations. You can only hunt geese from this month to this month. You can only fish from this hour to this hour. There's so many rules. I think that's why natives are frustrated, the Yupiks especially, and I think that's what's causing a lot of them to drink.

They're mad because they're not the hunter-warrior anymore and they beat up on their families and their wives. There's a lot of domestic violence and not taking care of their children and all that stuff. All their warrior-hunter spirit is gone because there's too many rules and regulations. They don't hunt anymore. They depend on the government too much.

I don't know how the hell that'll be ever solved. I think the white man's rules and regulations are here to stay. I think when our elders die, that's gonna be the end of the hunter-warrior spirit and all us younger natives are going to have to learn how to live the white man's way. Pretty soon we'll be only reading about how the Yupiks used to live and how they used to be hunters and warriors. Maybe we should start becoming white people and turn to the white man's way of life, then maybe we can lick this drinking problem.

I don't use drugs. I tried marijuana once but it made me too relaxed. I didn't like it. Everything got too slow. Everything was just weird. I never tried it again.

Drinking makes me feel, it just makes me feel *good*. I like to drink. That's the problem. I can't stop. (*laughs*) It makes me feel *good*. It makes me feel *relaxed*. It makes me *think*. It makes me feel really *high*. I haven't drunk in about two weeks and right now I'm all dried out and I feel *pretty good*.

I like being sober because a lot of my friends, they don't drink, and in order for me to go to visit them, I have to be sober. So if I want to keep my friends, if I want to go and visit them, I have to be sober. But I enjoy booze and I don't think I'll be sober *all* the time.

Yeah, I do have a drinking problem. I like the taste of booze and when I start, I can't stop. If I want to stop drinking, I can stop *for two weeks*. But to go *completely dry*, to *never, ever* drink again — I won't say that. I *can't say, I won't say*, that I will stop for ever and ever because I know I won't. I can't stop forever. I enjoy it too much.

5

ESCAPE
AND AFTERMATH

"I have two personalities. There's the person that's talking right now. I wouldn't hurt a flea. But there's also the other part of me, I call her the monster."

To Europeans and many other peoples, alcohol is regarded as a stimulating beverage meant to be taken in moderation to heighten the enjoyment of a meal or social occasion. Most native drinkers, however, have not yet learned how to use it that way. Instead, drinking is just the process they must go through to achieve the end they desire. Some people consciously sit down and drink to get drunk. Some drink to gain courage and lower inhibitions. But many drink to eliminate (temporarily) their worries and problems.

The rippling aftermath of excessive native drinking is felt in many different ways. The physical effects alone are horrendous because alcohol, after all, is poisonous and will kill if consumed in sufficient quantity. In addition to the physical effects, excessive drinking also has a devastating effect on an individual's attitude, behaviour and mental health. Worst of all, though, is the shattering effect that alcohol abuse has on non-drinking innocent people.

TUNGWENUK *is a twenty-nine-year-old Alaskan Inupiat. Muscular and clean-cut, he is breezy, self-assured and laughs loudly. He has been sober for three years.*

What did I like about drinking? Well, for one thing it was easier to pick up women. (*laughs*) It was easier to get laid. (*laughs*) It made throwing a pass at a woman a lot easier if the liquor was around. If it wasn't, it was really a strenuous activity to jump in the sack with a girl I was attracted to. I had a difficult time throwing passes at women when I wasn't drunk or I wasn't drinking. I think I was really self-conscious. I had a tremendous fear of associating with women and drinking gave me a false sense of security.

ALFRED *is the thirty-seven-year-old Cree who, in Chapter 4, described how he cheated a bootlegger out of a case of beer with a two-dollar bill. He is tall and thin with dark skin and a mop of thick black hair. He bears the marks of a long drinking career in northern Manitoba. His face is lopsided because one of his cheekbones has been kicked in.*

I got lots of scars from drinking. I even just about lost my eye. I had to go and have surgery in Winnipeg. It happened in The Pas, in a hotel room. I don't know who done it. I just woke up. I couldn't open my eyes. So they took me to Winnipeg. An emergency flight. That was two springs ago. Last summer I went back there to get bone grafting in my eye. It's better now. I was cross-eyed that time. They kicked in bone here (*points to his cheekbone*) and I had to get plastic surgery, they call it.

I got no teeth. All my teeth got kicked in. They were broken. They had to get pulled out. Now I need dentures. That's why I don't speak good. Everything seems to want to come whistling out when I talk. But once I get dentures, I'll be able to speak better. I hope.

That's what it has done to me, this alcohol.

D.L.S. is a thirty-seven-year-old Chippewa woman. She grew up in southern Ontario.

Drinking controlled me. I was driven by a madness that when I drank, I had to drink and drink and drink. But I never knew when I was gonna drink, it was so unpredictable. I acted out of impulse. I could be watching TV and see an advertisement of a cool glass with ice down the side and the next thing you know I would be on my way to the liquor store. I never knew what was gonna happen.

It interfered with every area of my life. I felt so estranged from my family, I would just hide and live in lies. My daughter is eighteen now, and she definitely has the effects of my life on her. She's very insecure and she's very vulnerable and very afraid. And it's affected her and my husband greatly. They have a hard time relating to me because I'm not predictable and I act impulsively. I try to dictate and control them and so on. It has devastated my family.

FRANK is a fifty-three-year-old Cayuga who grew up in southern Ontario. He speaks in a slow and deliberate monotone.

My worst hangover was actually beyond something that could be referred to as a hangover. I should have had medical help and once or twice I did go to the hospital for help. But the minute the nursing staff realized I was there for alcohol withdrawal, their attitude changed. I was like a moral outcast. It was very obvious that in spite of the fact that they were doing things for me, they were doing it reluctantly and with very little good will.

When I was sobering up, my nerves were bad. Even my thoughts could reduce me to tears — the old crying jag. (*sighs*) I was in a bad way. If I was awake, I was a wreck. When I finally did calm down enough to drop off to sleep, I would wake up choking, gasping for breath. I would be almost frantic sometimes.

Other times I would be in the bathroom holding onto the toilet bowl with the dry heaves, sweat running down my face. I would be so shaky that I could hardly remain standing. I was like a puppet on a string. My movements wouldn't even be co-ordinated. So in the sense that I had a hangover, I was beyond that.

RONBA is an attractive twenty-eight-year-old Manitoba Cree with a sly smile. For the past three months, she has been sober and undergoing treatment at Nelson House Medicine Lodge. She was interviewed there.

This one time I was drinking for two weeks straight and I tried to cure my hangover, so I tried drinking water. It didn't stay down. I'd keep throwing up. I tried juice, wouldn't stay down. Then I tried beer. Then I drank whiskey. Nope. Nothing would stay down. It felt like I was so dehydrated inside. So I just took little sips of water, probably about half a teaspoon, then I'd still be throwing up. I don't know where all that liquid came out from. Because I couldn't keep anything down.

About five o'clock in the afternoon, that's when I went into DTs [delirium tremens]. I seen a person right in front of my eyes, stirring something in his cup and I tried blocking my eyes, putting my fingers right in front of me. I couldn't get rid of him. I kept going, "Get away from me!"

I kept seeing that person in front of me and I kept on throwing up, so they took me to the hospital. They told my parents I was near death. Killing myself with booze. Poisoning myself. I stayed in the hospital five days. It went away that night. I thought it was getting better. It was on the third or fourth day I was in the hospital, it came back. But it was a different one. I was hearing my husband's voice. He was at work, an hour's drive away. I keep hearing his voice. I'd tell him, "What the hell are you doing here?" Like talking back to it? And he answers me? I thought I was going crazy. So the nurses stayed with me. I couldn't seem to get rid of him. I said, "Get out of here. Leave me alone."

It was scaring me to death. It finally went away about three hours later. I stayed in the hospital for another two days and signed myself out.

It's a very frightening experience for me, but I didn't learn my lesson. Stayed sober for two weeks. Went right back to the bottle. Still didn't learn nothing.

YVONNE is a thirty-one-year-old Cree from northern Alberta. She was interviewed in a native treatment centre. She has been sober for twenty-two days.

If I were sober I wouldn't jump into bed with just anybody but when I was drinking it didn't matter. I would go to bed with guys I normally wouldn't.

When I was eighteen, I had a boyfriend and I got angry at him for some reason, so I went to the bar. I met up with these guys and I went over to their trailer and I stayed there from Friday night to Sunday.

That first night I went to bed with this guy. The next day I got up, we started drinking again and I went with another guy. I ended up going to bed with about five guys that weekend. And it didn't matter to me. That's something I wouldn't do if I was sober. I don't think I'd even go to bed with even one of them if I had been sober. But I didn't care. I was just loose. I was just a piece of property.

You know, when I think back on it, I feel, oh, I feel dirty. Now it doesn't bother me as much 'cause I've learned to accept it. There's nothing I can do about it now, so what's the point of feeling bad?

WESLEY *is a dark-skinned, serious and slow-talking thirty-one-year-old from the Stoney reserve in southern Alberta.*

During my drinking days, this friend of mine got married to this woman, eh? She was drinking with him and they were only going out for a week and they got married.

This guy was daring for me to do that. So I was drinking in the bar and this lady came along, she was older than me, she was thirty-five at that time. I was drinking around with her for a week and I ended up marrying her. I married her because this friend dared me.

After I sobered up, realizing what I had done, I tried to

stick it out with her. I stuck it out for four years. But I couldn't handle it, so I got out of it.

I've been regretting doing that. Like, I never even cared about her. Was just a dare. Sometimes I feel guilty about it. I sort of feel I was using her. I wouldn't do that if I was sober, no way.

LINDA'S STORY

Linda is a twenty-five-year-old Dene from the Northwest Territories. She has baby-girl features and a soft, baby-girl voice. She has been sober for seven months.

Everybody that I knew growing up would drink a certain way. They were what is termed a binge alcoholic. They would sometimes go days, weeks, months without drinking and then suddenly they would have one drink and be drinking for weeks and months.

I remember a lot of fights. My dad would hit my mother and the whole family would get involved. My aunties would come over and they would be drinking and there would be big fights. I was scared. I was frightened. I just wished that they would stop.

Every time someone would drink in my family, they would have another personality come out and this personality would swear like I have never heard anybody swear before. If it was my mother it was "f" this, "f" that. Just such hate for the world. Such bitterness. And everything was just "fuck" and "shit." Everything. People were "bastards" and "bitches." That's all I can remember, the "f" word and "bitch." They would get so vicious. My mother would sit up at two in the morning and just curse the world. My uncles would do that.

My aunties would do that. My cousins would do it. Everyone that I saw getting drunk would end up with this anger.

I remember one time sleeping over at my auntie's house. My other aunt came home and she was drunk and she came into the bedroom and crawled into the next bed and she cursed all night. All night she cursed. She named people that may have done her wrong or had hurt her but all night, it was just one big fight for her. So that's the big impression I had about drinking as a young girl, that people got very angry and there was a lot of violence.

When Friday would come, my mother would prepare for her weekend drinking binges. She would clean up the whole house. The whole house was spotless. She would even buy us little gifts. You know, like new Barbie doll-clothes, that was the big thing. Or play food, the little boxes of cereal or whatever. She'd get the miniature size and get the little containers for us. And it would be a wonderful day. We'd come home on Friday and Mum was happy because the house was clean and, oh, we had these new toys. But that night my mum would start drinking. And if we'd say, "Oh, Mummy, don't go. Don't go drinking," she'd say, "Look. I've been working all week. I've cleaned this house for you. I've bought you these toys. Isn't that good enough for you? Aren't I a good enough mother for you? Goddammit."

And she'd march out the door only to come back at two in the morning with tons of people that she picked up at the dance or the bar. She'd blare the stereo, Hank Snow and Kitty Wells, full blast.

I started hating my mother, very much, and I would always question her drinking. I wanted to know, "Why do you drink? Why do you do this? Why?" You know, "Why?"

I don't know when it started exactly, I don't know what age, but my mum started picking on me. When everybody left from the party or if everyone passed out, there was my mother, her face distorted, nursing her bottle of beer. The record playing, maybe one or two lights, trying to smoke a cigarette. And then that anger and cursing the world would start.

But it wasn't just general cursing at everybody. It started to be on me.

"Linda's not my favourite," she would say. "Linda's not my favourite. Maryanne's my favourite. Maryanne does everything for me. Linda doesn't. Fucking Linda. Stupid bitch." Blah-blah-blah. You know?

I would sit up in my bed. I would lie awake for hours till she would finally conk out. And I would check to see if the cigarette was out. Sometimes I would bring a blanket for her and slowly put it over her. Praying that she wouldn't wake up. And then I would go to bed.

My mum decided that I was going to be her scapegoat. I was going to be the reason she was going to drink. So the way that I acted at home became very important. If I didn't do the dishes one night, or if I didn't bring in the clothes, or if I didn't iron my dad's shirts, or if I didn't play with Maryanne, my younger sister, then my mum would drink. She would find some way to twist that around so that she had a reason to drink. It was hard to live that way, always feeling that you were responsible for your mother's drinking.

When my mother would go out drinking, we would have a babysitter, and one of the babysitters we had was a cousin. I was about eight, I guess, and he was about fourteen, and he started sexually abusing me.

When it first happened, I didn't say anything. I dare not say anything to my mother, or my father or my sister or anybody. I didn't tell anybody. I kept it inside and I just sort of knew that it was a bad thing that had happened.

The next weekend she was wondering who to get to babysit. And I said, "Oh, no. Don't ask Sonny." And she said, "Why?"

And I said, "I don't really like him." And then she laid that whole bit on. "I do all this for you. Every day I do this. Don't ruin my chances of having one good night to myself. I deserve to go out with my friends. I've been looking after you all week."

And I would cry. I remember crying. I remember begging her and asking her not to have Sonny babysit. But she did and she went out drinking. So Sonny would come into the bedroom where me and Maryanne were sleeping. I remember trying to sleep right against the wall. I was on the top bunk. I was trying to keep as far away from him as I could, but he would always get me. Somehow I would get down and go with him. Once that was over, my mum would bring all her friends over and have a party.

I got drunk when I was twelve. I had so much anger at the age of twelve because of the things that happened to me. I got sick but I liked the state it put me in.

I was attracted to alcohol because it numbed me. It gave me permission to swear and it also gave me permission to be a bitch. It gave me permission to raise hell if I wanted to and scream out that anger. And I did. I did. I was only twelve. (*laughs*) I can't believe that now. I started smoking. I started swearing. I started drinking and I started hanging around with an older crowd.

A big change in my life was when I came to Yellowknife. In Inuvik, the classes in school were fifty-fifty aboriginal peoples — there were Gwich'in, some Slavey, the Inuvialuit, some Inuit from Keewatin and the rest were white students. I never felt threatened in that way.

But when I came to Yellowknife, the school I went to was predominantly white. I was threatened a little bit. I felt uncomfortable. I remember a couple of boys behind me as I was walking home going, " Squaw. Squaw. Squaw. Squaw."

When I enrolled in the English and social studies and math courses, there were hardly any native students. I was sometimes the only one. The attitude of the white students was, "All Indians are drunks." They didn't call 'em *Dene*. They called 'em *Indians* and *drunks*. Part of me believed it, because all the adults in my family drank. And they didn't drink like a drink or two and everybody went home, they drank and they drank and they drank until someone got hurt or until there was no more booze to be had.

In school I wouldn't sit up in my chair. I slowly withdrew. I rarely asked questions. If I did I was afraid of what I might say and I wanted to be very, very careful because I wasn't strong enough to defend native people and to stand up for who I was and what I believed in. I couldn't do it. I wasn't strong enough. And that made me mad. I was angry at myself for not being that strong. I wanted so much to believe in who I was that it just seemed when the weekends would come my mother would drink and call me every name in the book so I had no self-esteem, no self-confidence.

The times I did have it, I was drinking. Or a boy found me attractive. So those were the ways that I felt good about myself — through drinking and physical attraction. That's all I thought I had to offer anybody. Not too good.

I didn't do very well in high school. I didn't do as well as I could have. I did well in math, very well. And the reason was because there were no social problems raised in math. No main characters came into conflict with other characters over racial themes. They were just numbers. Everybody was equal. I wasn't afraid to go up to the board and isolate an integer or whatever. I did it and it was easy for me. But all the other subjects — social studies, English, psychology, I didn't do very well.

I cared more when I was a teenager. Even as a child I cared more. I was more sensitive than anybody else. When my friends had a problem, with their mother or their father or their boyfriend or whatever, I sat and I listened and maybe that story was boring as hell, but I sat there and listened. And I probably heard that story ten times already anyway, but I sat there and I listened and I cared and I worried about them. But when I tried to talk about what was happening in my life, I never had anybody. There was never anybody there to listen to me. Never.

It may have been that time where I *split*. I realized in the last couple months that I have two personalities. There's the person that's talking right now. I wouldn't hurt a flea. I wouldn't squish a spider. The way that I am right now. But there's also the other part of me, who's very vicious. Very mean. Very loud. Aggressive. Obnoxious. Rude. And very, very angry. I call her the monster. I went to a counsellor and I said, "There's this part of me that I don't really like."

I described it as a monster and she said, "What does it look like?"

I turned to the right of me and I saw this person who looked like me but who just had this growl in her. Her face was all distorted as if ready to kill. And it just made me cry.

I think the monster part of me is probably not as big as I believe. I'm exploring the idea that she may be an angry, confused, hurt little girl if you take away that anger. But she's developed a shield, maybe a mask. I don't know, it's so new to me now.

I'm involved in a relationship and have been for the last four years. It's a good relationship. It's growing. I've made a commitment to deal with my issues and I've made a commitment to grow and Tom has decided to stand beside me.

One time Tom and I started an argument and it blew up to be a huge verbal fight. Arguing back and forth. And the monster came. Bang. And I just reamed Tom up and down. I just cursed him. I did everything to break him and I did break him. I hurt him so badly. I told him to get out of my life. Leave. Now. And I kept repeating that I hated him. I hated him so much for taking away some responsibility that I thought should have been mine, or whatever. Tom left and slowly I came down from that monster character. I cried and took a deep breath and wondered where Tom was and if he would come home. He came home and I said I was sorry. And then about two days after we were talking again, Tom said, "Well, I sure don't want to see another fight like that."

And I said, "What fight? What do you mean?"

Honest to goodness, I totally forgot about it! Here was something that had devastated him and to me it was like, "What fight? I don't remember."

It was at that point that I realized I've got a lot of work to do on that monster part of me. That monster part of me probably saved my life in a lot of circumstances when I was growing up. It probably did. But I'm not as threatened as I was when I was a child anymore and I have to learn to deal with that monster part in me.

Right now my life is almost chaotic. I've stirred up a lot of things in my memory and I realize the ways I do things are new and they are different. I'm scared a lot of times. It's all new territory for me and I always want to fall back into my old habits and negative feelings. You know, just sort of plop back in it because it's so damn comfortable, eh? It's the way I grew up and it's the way I survived. But I know that I can't live like that anymore. I have to change.

I don't resent my parents anymore. I love my mum and dad. I realize they did the best they could. My dad's mother died when he was about four. He was forced to be put in a hostel in Fort Chipewyan when he was about five and he grew up in a hostel. So my dad had no idea how to be a father, you know?

My mum grew up like that. Both her parents are alcoholics. She also had tuberculosis from the age of twelve to twenty-one, and she grew up in a hospital with nurses and doctors poking her all the time.

So I've been able to look at them as human beings. They're sick and they're alcoholic. And bad things happened when I grew up. But I'm learning to deal with them and the anger I feel towards my mum and dad lessens every day. It's turning into love, a deeper and fuller love than I ever had felt for them before.

All my life I've learned practical things. I've learned that if I eat too much I'm going to get fat. If I don't eat I'll fade away. I've learned that exercise is good. I've learned how to take care of my body physically.

I know about education, going to school, getting a diploma, going on to university, getting a good job, feeding your mind with information. Taking care of myself mentally.

Things that I didn't really consider were how to nurture my spirit and how to nurture the emotional part of me. I usually felt two things. I felt happy and I felt angry. Those were really the only two kinds of emotions I ever felt. For the longest time I would bounce back and forth. I had blocked out feeling sad. I had blocked out all the other types of emotions I could have into feeling good and feeling angry. So I had a lot of emotional growing to do and I had a lot of spiritual growing to do. And I still have a lot of spiritual and emotional growing to do today. I'm just at the tip of the iceberg in that department.

I'm dealing with a lot of the anger, frustrations, fear, confusion that I felt as a child because of my parents' drinking. I've learned a lot of patterns of behaviour that are unhealthy. I don't know how to deal with anger when it comes up to me and when that monster flares up. I'm learning now how to deal with that in a healthy way. At the same time I'm building up my confidence in myself as a Dene.

The beliefs of native people are so relevant today and are so meaningful. I'm building back some of that pride. I think that alcohol took a lot of that pride away from me.

I don't drink anymore. I have two boys: they'll soon be five and three. I don't want to pass on that cycle, so I decided not to drink. I made the decision not to drink just seven months ago but before that I was slowly cutting back and slowly looking at myself when I drank. I didn't want to end up like my mother and I found that even if I had one or three drinks it wasn't satisfying.

I was at a spiritual gathering in Fort Simpson in August in '89. An elder spoke about alcohol and the drastic things that have happened to native people because of it. He talked about when people drink, they chase their spirit away, even if they have just one tablespoon. They've put that into the blood and they've offset the balance in the body and the connection that the blood in our body has with Mother Earth and Father Sky.

I thought about that. I looked out on the Deh Cho [Mackenzie River] and I thought about it for a long time and it made sense to me. Maybe it's sort of a simple way of looking at things, but it made sense to me. The elder also went on to say that without that spirit, you become jealous. You become a different person and you're very vulnerable to other things. I made the decision at that gathering not to drink again. And I haven't. And I can feel my spirit getting stronger.

6

CRAZINESS

"Please gimme some more dope. Please gimme some more dope. I'll do anything for you if you gimme some more dope."

The Stoney people and the Ojibway people knew what they were talking about when they named wine and alcohol "crazywater" in their languages because people do many crazy things under its influence. The craziness ranges from bizarre and inexplicable behaviour to the outer reaches of insanity.

ELSTON is an eighteen-year-old Stoney from southern Alberta. He's tall, skinny and has a punky, new-wave haircut. Elston is a talented sketch artist. He's also good with a yo-yo. He began drinking heavily when he was twelve.

One time me and my cousin and my brother were drinking out in the forest. My brother kind of got rowdy and hit me. I hit him back and I kicked him in the face. He went down and I sat on him and just punched on his face, punching away. He throw me back and he jumped on me, hitting me. My cousin got up and kicked my brother in the ribs. He fall back and my cousin was just kicking him.

My brother was wearing boots and he kicked my cousin in the balls and he went down and he couldn't fight. So I fought with him, eh? I was blacked out and the next thing I remember, I was on the ground, on my face, and he was on my back, grabbing my hair, holding my head up and he was saying, "Who's the toughest?"

I didn't answer and he hit me in the face and he told me, "Who's the toughest?" He kept hitting me in the face and I didn't answer. Every time I don't answer, he kept hitting me in the face. And I told him, "It's you. You're the toughest."

Then my cousin got up and kicked my brother in the head. He went down and I got up and I kicked him in the face and kicked him in the ribs. I told my cousin to get out of the way and I grab a wood about this thick (*spreads his hands a foot apart*) and I lift it up and I drop it in his stomach. My cousin kick him in the nose and broke his nose. My cousin told him, "Next time I'm not gonna be so nice."

My face was just all swollen up. My lips were popped out. I had black eyes. The left eye, I can hardly open it. And I had a broken nose at the time. All beat up. My cousin the same thing. My brother the same thing. And he had both side of broken ribs 'cause I dropped that tree on him.

I blacked out and the next thing I remember I was with my brother, drinking again — after I fight with him. Just sitting on top of a hill drinking with him again.

SUE is a thirty-one-year-old Metis from southern Manitoba. She has a matter-of-fact attitude and calls herself a social drinker.

My mother died because of alcohol. She was bludgeoned to death when I was about five. She used to drink quite a bit. She was only thirty-three and had four kids and was living on welfare in the north end of Winnipeg at the time. She used to like to drink and party. One night, one of her boyfriends, they were drinking and she was passed out in the bed, he just bludgeoned her to death with a gun and in the morning we got up and found her there.

She used to drink a lot and the people she drank with were all very heavy drinkers and abusive people. So if that's the type of lifestyle you choose for yourself, that's what will happen. Unfortunately, it happened to her. She was with the wrong person, I guess. She lived in an abusive environment and she just never seemed to get away from it. You know, she attracted those type of people. It hasn't changed my attitude toward drinking or anything. I don't know why it hasn't, but it hasn't.

WALTER is half Cree and half Assiniboine and comes from Saskatchewan. He is thirty-six years old, short, dark and tough-looking. He has been sober for eighteen days and is on a waiting list to enter a public treatment program. He was interviewed in an outdoor Calgary mall.

My girlfriend and I had been partying all night over at the village. We were heading home and as we were rounding this corner I could see there was a car coming from our place, so my girlfriend says, "That looks like your friend Barry."

And I says, "Yeah, that's their station wagon." He was a good friend of mine.

They start flashing their lights indicating for us to stop. So I pulled over and he gets out and he says, "Hi. How ya' doing?"

I'm pretty damn drunk and I says, "Oh, I'm doin' all right. I'm just heading home."

And he says, "Oh, I was wondering if I could borrow twenty dollars. I'll pay you back next week."

I says, "I'm sorry. I don't have any money. My old lady's got it all."

So he walks around to the side of my truck and he opens the door and punches her out. He didn't even ask her anything. He just nails her. And you could tell her nose was broke just by the sound of the crunch, eh? Blood's flying all over.

His nephews jumped out. There must have been three or four of them. They all jumped out, so I figure it's time to get out of here. So I grabbed onto my girlfriend's arm and I put the truck into low and I just took off and he was still trying to hang onto the door but he had to let go 'cause it was taking off too fast. We got to the top of the hill and she says, "Honey, aren't you gonna do anything about this?"

And I says, "Well, hand me that gun. I'll go back after them."

So while I was racing down the hill after them trying to see where they're going, she reaches inside the glove compartment and she stuck a bullet in the chamber of the .22. They were just coming from the service station. They were coming towards me and I pulled in front of them to block them. I jumped out with my .22. It was loaded but I didn't know it. I pointed the gun at Barry and I told him, "You fuckin' woman fighter." I tol' him. "How come you hit my ol' lady?"

And he says, "You don't have enough guts to pull that trigger."

So I tol' him, "Well, watch me."

It surprised the hell out of me when that gun fired. It just killed him instantly. That sort of sobered me up. So I phoned the police and an ambulance and I waited right there. He had already died in the meantime and I told the cops everything that happened.

As I thought about it later in the cells, it seemed like a bad dream, something you'd dream about, eh? But I woke up and I looked and there's the bars. I couldn't believe it, so I called one of the cops over and I says, "And what am I charged with?"

He says, "You're charged with second-degree murder."

It just shocked me that I had taken a life. I never would have did this if I was sober, eh? 'Cause of my training in the armed forces. Never to point a weapon at anyone, eh? Unless you mean to use it. But I was so drunk that I didn't see her putting the shell in the gun.

When I went to court I told them I wanted to plead guilty to a lesser charge. So they said, "Okay, manslaughter."

So these are things I look back on, you know, with remorse. I used to have bad dreams about that, eh? I guess anyone with a conscience would. This is all works of the devil I guess.

Alcohol. Just drags a man down so bad, so far, so fast.

DIANE'S STORY

Diane is a thirty-six-year-old Tlingit from the Alaska panhandle. Despite years of hard living and traumatic abuse, she looks barely half her age. She is an actress and playwright with the striking looks and the tall, thin bearing of a model. Diane has been clean and sober for five years. She was interviewed in an Anchorage hotel room.

My parents got divorced when I was three. My mom left the state and my dad sort of tried to take care of us, but he was a gambler and a drinker and just couldn't do it. I got put in a lot of foster homes. I couldn't count the number.

I was five years old and I remember being without food and my brothers and I sleeping on plywood in an attic. These white people wouldn't feed us and they would really torment us. I would be too scared to ask for a piece of bread because of what they would do. We wanted to get in an Indian foster home, but the State wouldn't let us do that. They had the attitude that Indians would have too much alcohol, which is really ironic because the foster homes I lived in were disgusting.

Eventually we lived with this older white lady outside of Ketchikan. We lived near the pulp mill, and that stunk. We lived subsistence, getting clams and fish from the water where we lived. We knew what it was like to live poor. We used to get our bedding and stuff out of the garbage dump. We would go shopping at the garbage dump.

She took care of us best way she knew how but she had a sick family that really drank a lot. She had grandkids that were really abusive.

I moved in with them when I was six and I stayed with them until I was fifteen. I was sexually abused a lot in that home. It was real sick. Her grandson was the one and there was a lot of denial in the family that it was happening. There was no one to talk to about it and I felt like I was living in a *nightmare*.

We lived with a lot of prejudice too. There was so much prejudice then. Every day in every way we were told we were nobody. It didn't matter if you were light-skinned Indian or dark-skinned Indian, (*cries*) as long as you were Indian, you were less.

Getting beat up on the school bus was getting pretty old and the bus driver not doing nothing while the kids take you down in the back and punch your face in. You know, having my lunch thrown on the floor and having my face pushed into the wall and getting a bloody nose. They thought it was pretty funny. And they'd say that us Indians stank and we smelt like fish and so many names, you know — "fish-crunchers" and all this stuff.

One day this one white girl I shared a locker with in junior high came up and said, "I can't run around with you anymore because my boyfriend doesn't like Indians."

And for some reason, something just snapped inside of me. "That's the last straw. That's *it*."

I just felt this big surge of *hate* and *rage* and *anger* like I had never felt in my life. I had done so much to follow the Bible and turn the other cheek and pray for your enemies and on and on and on and at that moment I decided it was all a lie. And in one day I *changed*.

I was twelve years old then and I made a serious decision to go get drunk. I went and stole a bottle from this bar up the road from where we lived. And I went home and hid in my room and I drank a whole fifth of Calvert's Extra by myself.

I woke up in a pool of vomit. I couldn't hold food down for several days. I was close to dying from alcohol poisoning. I tried to go to school and I threw up in school, on the bus. I was *really* sick.

They had the police out at the house investigating the stolen booze and they found an empty bottle underneath my dresser. The police showed up and I go out the window, off and running. That was the first time I ran away but the police found me.

When I was eleven, twelve, thirteen, fourteen, all I ever wanted was my mother. And that was just never gonna happen. Matter of fact, when I ran away from home I thought somehow that would make her come. I was wrong. I went to jail. (*laughs*) I spent my first night in jail for stealing a blanket to stay warm. So I was a big criminal and for the first time the white kids weren't beatin' me up on the school bus 'cause they were afraid of me. I had mixed feelings about that. First I felt kind of sad about it and then I immediately after felt like, "Good. Now at least I know what I am."

I was very, very angry by the time I was twelve years old. I would get busted for curfew violations and smoking and stealing liquor. I would sit under the boardwalks in Ketchikan with a bottle of wine and wish I would die. I think I started death-wishing when I was eleven or twelve. Sometimes I would cut myself up with a razor on my wrists and wish I could cut right through. I did that a lot.

I used drugs and alcohol heavily when I was twelve and thirteen and fourteen and fifteen. *Anything* I could put into my system that might alter me I would take it. I would sniff any kind of inhalant from gas to Pam to fingernail cleaner to paint. Anything. I was deep into an alcohol problem and on uppers really bad.

And then I lost one of my best friends. He gave me a beaded necklace that his mom gave to him and I still have it. He died on the streets from overdosing and drinking. I was with him and I knew he was gonna die. (*sighs*) We lost a lot of people. We lost lots of people to suicide. When I was a teenager I thought there was nothing but death and pain in the world, so I drank and used to make the pain go away. When I drank I just didn't want to feel anything.

While I was in junior high one time I ran away from home and a bunch of other kids decided to go with me. We were all Indian except for the two white girls that were part of our gang. We broke into the old hospital and stayed in the boiler room. We were camping in there for a week and we did all kinds of different things to get booze and food.

Then the cops found us and they burst through the door. I always remember that 'cause I was thirteen at the time and there was a ten-year-old boy sitting next to me. They burst through that door and I *jumped*, man, because it was that startling. A cop's gun came into my face and he held it on me and he said, "You make one fucking move and I'll blow your head off."

And all I could think was, "I'm thirteen years old and I have a cop's gun in my face and there's this ten-year-old kid sitting next to me."

They hauled us off to jail. We had *piles* of charges against us — breaking and entering, destruction of government property, minors in possession, on and on and on.

I got arrested not long after that for assault with a deadly weapon against a white girl. We were really into switchblades then. I went to court and I ended up getting put back on probation. It's hard to remember all the arrests because they were rather frequent for a couple years there. I learned to act real tough, like I didn't need anybody. I would always feel successful when people would tell me I was intimidating.

I ran away so many times I can't count. Metlakatla is a Tsimshian reservation right next door to Ketchikan. I used to go over there and hide out 'cause it was all Indian people and we would feel at home, you know, but the state troopers came and hauled us out of there. They made me go to the children's home in Ketchikan.

When I was fourteen, the president of the senior class invited me out on a date and this is where I really learned something about my drinking. This was like my first *date* instead of just hanging out with the guys and everything.

My foster parent sewed me a dress instead of getting something from the Salvation Army. And it was real nice. He came to pick me up and I was all nervous and everything. He was *somebody* and he belonged to a family of somebodies and he was this *white* guy and everything.

And he says he's got to stop up at his parents' apartment. There was nobody there and his parents are gone for the weekend as it turns out. And the next thing I know, he's trying to rip my clothes off and shit. I'm rather tough at the time and I was punching him out as much as he was trying to get me down. This guy ain't gonna let me go and I'm scared and I'm *angry*. I knocked him to the floor a couple of times. And then there was a knock at the door and then these buddies come in. I mean what kind of a set-up is this? It's pretty damn apparent. Let's gang-bang the little Indian girl for a good time. It's like this is the status we have here.

God, I could kill them, even still. And they bring out the tequila. "Let's have a party." So I *drank* because I'm either gonna drink till I don't feel anything regardless of what happens or I'm gonna drink until *they* are too drunk. But one way or another I'm gonna be drunk. I don't know how much tequila we killed off, but those guys passed out and I drank every damn one of them under the table. I left there having bruises from fighting them off and all the *grabbing* and the *pinching*. I went home and I went to the burn barrel outside the house and I put the dress in it and I burned it. And when my foster parent asked me the next morning how was my date I told her, "It was fine," 'cause I just couldn't tell her the truth.

I had a real hard time with white men and white people after that. I was really, really, *really* full of hatred. I *hated* them so much. I hated *everything* they ever did to me. (*punches her hand*) I hated *everything* they did to divide up my people and take my brothers away. *Everything*. I hated them. It's taken *all* of my adult life to this point to get rid of that hatred that was crippling me. And I would drink and get *utterly* belligerent.

And I was really wretchedly lonely. All through my twenties. I *blew* my twenties to hell. My twenties was completely nothing but drugs and alcohol and that's all it was. I mean I tried to hold *jobs*. I got pregnant and had a *kid*. But I used all that stuff about being enraged about prejudice, all this violence, all this *anger*, all this *injustice* and somehow it became a convenient excuse to destroy myself.

When I was fifteen, my foster parent died one morning and I found her body. So I left that day for Metlakatla and I went to my boyfriend's house. That night he got drunk and I got drunk and the parents got drunk. And then they got in a fight and the windows got broken and the glass was flyin' and the blood was sprayin' everywhere. The kids were screamin'.

So I made them stop. I told the parents to quit fighting. I made them get Lyle to the hospital. I made the kids go to bed. I was just in control. (*laughs nervously*) The blood was all over and I mopped it up. I was wringing out mopfuls of blood. And after everything was taken care of, I sat down with a fifth and I drank it like water.

And when Lyle came home I sat up with him the rest of the night because he was in such pain 'cause he lost flesh out of his hand.

I stayed up till the sun came up and then I heard gunshots across the street and the folks next door, well, the dad, he shot himself in front of his family. (*cries*) That's what alcohol does to our people. (*cries*) I don't talk about that day too much. I used to joke that that was just a very bad day.

When my foster parent died, my brother and I ran away to Metlakatla but the state troopers brought us back and put us in another foster home. Finally, they shipped me off to Sitka to stay with my grandparents because I'd been kicked out of Ketchikan High 'cause I drank and vandalized the school. The principal told me I was the worst kid he had seen in nineteen years of being around schools. (*laughs*)

I was supposed to go to Mount Edgecumbe Indian Boarding School. I remember living on the streets and getting loaded and having a good old happy time. Me and my girlfriends who were Indian made this big plan that we were gonna run away. So I tied a bunch of blankets together and hustled out the second-storey window of my grandmother's house. I couldn't get the blankets back in the window, so they were just hanging out the window. I ran out to the ferry and the police arrested us out there. There was a *big* stink all over town about the fact that I had the blankets hanging out the window. No one ever forgot that, even to this day.

So I went to the city jail in Sitka. In those days you got arrested for running away. They didn't have juvenile facilities in Sitka, so you just went to the city jail. It wasn't the first time I stayed in jail without any charges, without a hearing, without anything.

I spent two weeks in jail. It was like something out of a western, you know. You got bars from the ceiling to the floor. They came in and they took the mattress away. They took the toothbrush, anything that was loose in the cell, they took away. I laid down on the floor. I was just freezing. Everything was just metal and concrete, you know, and I was cold and I used my cowboy boots for a pillow and that's when they came and took *those* away.

I got out of jail because it was time to go to school. Time to go to school. (*laughs*) And I thought, "This is great 'cause this is gonna be a new school and I'm gonna get to start a new life and that'll be nice." (*laughs*) But the police escorted me to school in handcuffs. I'm in my jeans and these cowboy boots that I had been wearing in jail for two weeks. So everybody's like checking this out, right? "Look! Look at this person getting out of a police car, in handcuffs, going to school!"

It's hard to act like you got anything to offer when you got a cop standing next to you and you just got out of jail. How can I start fresh when I get that kind of reputation right off the bat? Actually, I did sort of start a new life. I actually became a halfway decent student at Mount Edgecumbe. I went to school, finished the year, did good and really thought I might do something with my life.

I was tryin' not to drink then. I decided I was gonna be a good student and everything. I was really tryin' to do good. A part of me always wanted to be something, be somebody, do something. I got out of the whole gang mode and out of the excessive drinking and drugging. I made it into honour dorm at school, but I'd sneak out and go get loaded. I wasn't *that* away from drugs and alcohol. And that's when I really started to get into mescaline and acid and mushrooms. The school tried to say that I was the first one to introduce hallucinogenics to the school. I don't think that's true but I don't know.

I graduated from high school in Fairbanks and I got kicked out of that foster home the next day 'cause they were like, "Our time with you is up. We no longer have any commitment to you. Out of here."

And no one was there at the graduation that I knew. No family, no foster family, nobody who could give a shit that Diane graduated from school. I was feeling pretty sorry for myself. I had no place to go, so I hit the road. I went to the States. I met Hell's Angels and other bikers and I was havin' a ball. I was goin' to concerts and pow-wows. I was drinkin' whiskey and smoking pot and doin' hash. That was the first time I did any heroin. I didn't really know what it was and I threw up a lot at first, but I liked it. I did that whole trip for a year. And it felt like everything was about *peace* and everything was about *love* and everything was about getting very loaded.

Fighting the war was like I was somebody. But I sure didn't have any morale or any self-respect. I tried selling drugs and I was so bad at it that I decided that I'd only get arrested, so I decided to drop that whole scene. I tried to prostitute myself to get some money but I didn't know what I was doin' so I didn't go through with it.

I started to drink again, I mean like really staring at the bottom of that bottle after that. Life was ugly. At nineteen years of age, I felt old. I felt old and I felt used up.

I got myself into the university then, but I screwed it all up. I never got any passing grades.

But I got a job at Fairbanks Native Association and I also won Miss Fairbanks Native Association. I was the *queen* for a year. Some queen. I was really trying to do a good job. There was a bunch of Indian women being killed in Fairbanks at that time and nobody was doing anything about it. Seven Indian women disappeared, so we started organizing self-defence for Indian women and walk the streets in pairs and don't go anywhere alone and this kind of stuff.

I went to a town meeting where I brought native people to the city council and I mean I made a big ruckus. I flew to San Diego for FNA to represent the National Congress of American Indians. And I went to Juneau to work on some mental health thing and I was just *doin'* stuff.

I was one of the youngest people to serve on the Fairbanks Native Association's executive board, I mean I was just jumping along, right? Bam, bam, bam. And I was (*snorts*) their drug and alcohol counsellor. I'm nineteen years old trying to counsel people who have lost their sister or their daughter because somebody murdered them and mangled them and left their body on the highway. But I couldn't handle it. I didn't have none of that shit straightened out in my own head. I don't have the skills. I don't have the training. And I finally can't take it. One day something snapped inside. I walked out and went down to the riverbank and sat down with one old guy and one middle-aged guy who spent their lives drinking. I sat down with them and knew that's where I belonged. We sat there all afternoon and got shitfaced.

So I decided to go work on the pipeline. I signed up with the union, paid my dues, went home, packed up my stuff, walked out and went to work.

The pipeline is where I met cocaine. And whiskey and cocaine became my life for the next three years. Everything was about drugs and booze. We'd play cards for grams and for bottles. I didn't work unless I was loaded. I was a truck driver and I packed two or three bottles and a quarter-ounce of coke to get me through a run. (*laughs*) It's amazing that pipeline ever got built. Those days, in the middle seventies, I was making up to $1,000 a week take-home and it's all just going up the nose and down the throat and in the arm.

I couldn't go a day without coke and whiskey. I *couldn't* make it a day, the shakes would get so bad. I had a journal I was writing in about this and I was pleading just to make it through the day. Just to make it through the comin' down.

I went on an "R and R" [rest and relaxation] to Arizona. I'd been drinking in this bar and I'd had women tell me you should probably watch out for this guy I'd seen. But when I seen him in the parking lot, he says, "Hey, can you help me?" So I rolled down the window. Next thing I know I got a knife at my throat and I got taken on a little drive. Rape — at knifepoint. It was brutal. This time by an Indian man. The man passed out in my car and the cops arrested him. They took me to the hospital and I'd been beat up by this guy and I was hurtin'.

I decided that would certainly have to be the last time this shit was gonna happen. It certainly shattered my image of the *Indian* man, which I think I probably blew out of proportion because of all the anger and hatred that I had towards white people and the stuff that they had done to me. I mean, what am I going to do now? Hate *everybody*? I couldn't hate all men. My brothers were all men, my dad was a man. I loved them. But it certainly put another wrinkle into things, I'll tell you that.

And when I went back to the pipeline, I started shooting dope. I knew one thing was certain. I didn't want to *feel* anything. I didn't want to feel anything in my *head*. I didn't want to feel anything *physically*. I didn't want to feel *nothin'*. I had somewhat of a promiscuous side to me with all the confusion around sex but I wanted somehow to have some integrity with it. Like the *one* thing that I could hang onto was somehow if I could just protect myself *sexually* I would be okay. And that just didn't seem to happen.

Fairbanks turned into a real horror town with the pipeline, it really did. Some friends were shot at by white people and then some white guy chased down this bunch of girls that I knew and rammed his pickup into their car and killed a girl. And nobody did *anything*. He was from a prominent white family, right? And that's all that seemed to matter. Indian people were getting killed and brutalized and it was like a misdemeanour.

We lost a lot of people. (*sighs*) Once I had this boyfriend who lived in the village. We met in a bar. I thought he was pretty neat; he raced dogs and everything. But he got drunk and shot himself. I think that's what pushed me over the edge. I tried many times in my adult life to quit drinking and using and I just couldn't do it. It just seemed that when he died, I gave up. I would try to get off the dope and try to get off the booze and I just couldn't seem to do it. I'd make promises with myself, I'd make bets with myself. I'd make bets with my friends. I'd make bets with my family. I would try to ac' like I was sober in public during the day and I would go home and drink at night.

It was a pretty degrading environment all the way around. I had enough money to keep myself loaded. Then the pipeline was over and I had a very expensive cocaine habit and an alcohol habit that wouldn't quit. And I didn't have any income. So I'd sell some dope or whatever to keep myself goin'. And I would do speed instead of coke and I would drink beer instead of expensive whiskies to keep the budget down, you know.

I started doing some work with the elitists of town, I got a job with the AFN, Alaska Federation of Natives. I started learning about wine, like from the wine books and how to order wine for dinner. I figured if I learned how to drink that way I wouldn't have a problem. So I started learning about Pooey-Foomay or whatever the hell the stuff was instead of Boone's Farm one month old. I ended up in Hawaii with an elitist in a fancy, fancy condo. Rollin' in the dough and rollin' in everything and sneaking off from that so I could get loaded and roll in something else. Really went off on a binge over there. Major binge.

I was tootin' heroin and tootin' coke and free-basin' coke and doin' quaaludes and doin' martinis, Tanqueray martinis, of course — straight up with a lemon twist — and all of this kind of crap. But it was cool. I was really cool. Sure.

I quit working for AFN after I came back and I got little jobs here and there. I even pumped gas. I was partyin' here and partyin' there. But it wasn't the same because we didn't have hundred-dollar bills to toot up our coke with. We had one-dollar bills with cross-tops — speed. It just wasn't the same. Real cheap stuff and it was getting sleazier by the day. I'd crush up cross-tops and toot — and God, that burns your nose.

Then I got pregnant and the only thing I was grateful for was that his Dad was Indian. And for the first time I got 98 percent off of drugs and alcohol, cigarettes, coffee and everything while I was pregnant. I knew that whatever I did affected this baby and I didn't want that. I didn't know a damn thing about babies, and I didn't even like babies, but I was real fascinated by something that was growing inside of me.

And when he was born, I thought I *have* to become somebody. I have to not be worthless. I can't be the angry tough guy anymore. I saw his face and I wanted to be a mother, whatever that was. I wanted to be somethin' special. I wanted this little person to look up at me. I was real ignorant about babies. It's amazing he made it through babyhood. (*laughs*) I dropped him in a little bag and carried him around like potatoes. I just didn't know what you're supposed to do. (*laughs*)

But I had terrible rages. I had a terrible temper. I would do terrible things in the bars and scream at white people and kick tables over and threaten people and smash things and vandalize and I didn't think anything of it. If somebody said something to me in a bar I didn't like, I'd pick them up by the *throat*. Of course, I used to pick up hundred-pound barrels from driving trucks. I was prone to extreme outrageous outbursts. But there's something about a baby screamin' in a crib while you're throwin' a temper that kind of goes, "Maybe you need to change your behaviour and find some help," 'cause it ain't cool to scare a baby. Some little thing had ticked me off and I smashed the coffee table, smashed a camera and just started smashing things. I'm going, "*God*. What am I *doing*?" And the baby's crying away in the crib. I went to the phone and I called the crisis line.

I started gettin' therapy for my rages. But I would *lie*. I would lie to every single therapist 'cause they would always ask, "Do you drink?"

"No. I don't drink. Well, very little. Nothing significant."

"Do you do drugs?"

"No, never." Talk about lie.

I stopped breastfeeding my son after three months 'cause I wanted to get *on* with it. I wanted to be able to drink again. I thought I could just do a casual gram here and there. I could have a few beers here and there. And it didn't work that way. It didn't work that way at all. I started leavin' him at my cousin's and I started pretendin' that the partyin' they were doin' wasn't takin' place. I felt that I was doin' the responsible thing if I said to her, "Now you guys don't party tonight while you have the baby here." Like that's gonna stop it. And I say I'm gonna be back probably around midnight and I show up three and a half days later.

I was going to college and I wanted somehow to be something, to be somebody. For exams I was just crammin' down drugs like crazy and takin' vitamins on top of it because I figured it would balance it out somehow. I had myself all convinced I was doin' the healthy thing, (*laughs*) takin' Vitamin B all night long, along with cross-tops and coke and beer to wash everything down.

I became a real Dr. Jekyll and Mr. Hyde in my last few years of using. I really wanted to look responsible and I didn't want anyone to threaten me with takin' my kid away.

I made it through school. I graduated in '85, amazingly enough. By that time I had so many three-day weekends I couldn't remember and the ones I could remember were so humiliating and so devastating that I couldn't face myself in the mirror. God, the life-and-death situations I put myself in with ex-cons I would pick up somewhere who had some dope and who were anxious to have some fun and I would give it to 'em. And I wouldn't remember shit except that I'd be sick, bruised, miserable. And what I could remember was just so awful. I'd be so disgusted I hated that person in the mirror. She was a slob. She was a slut. She was a nobody.

And I got into self-abuse again. Only worse. Pullin' my hair out till my head bled. Scratching my arms and my body and my legs until they would bruise or bleed. Hitting myself. Banging my head into a wall until I had bruises on my head or lumps. Biting myself until I punctured the skin or I couldn't take the pain anymore. It's like so much self-loathing. Just incredible intense self-hatred. I would tie things around my neck and try to hang myself and it wouldn't work and I'd get so mad and I didn't know how to do it right. And I would start overdosing on drugs really bad. I would convulse and veins would feel like they're popping out of my skull and my neck and everything. That was very painful. And I would just go on convulsing and I had no control of my body. I would come to and everything would be just numb on my left side and I would be groping around. I started getting extremely, extremely paranoid. I would crawl around floors at night thinking somebody was trying to kill me. I would lay in bed sometime with DTs so bad that rats were running out of the vents and up over the bed and up the bedposts and crawling under the covers and I would be screaming and slapping at everything. I would have trouble breathing and the physical reactions just got worse each time I used.

Somewhere I crossed the line and I entered a real dark and gloomy place where no matter how desperately I tried, the high never got good. It never got good again. I needed to have more of everything and it just wasn't working. The noise wouldn't stop in my head and my skin was making me crazy. It was like I wanted to rip my skin off. Sometimes I would wake up with bruises up and down my legs and my hips 'cause I'm tryin' to pull my skin off and everything. And just feeling nuts and out of my mind.

I was out of my mind. I'd be up in the night crawling around the bathroom floor, just rolling around in pain from any momentary withdrawal. And I'd have to get loaded again. "I got to get to the liquor store and it'll get me until I can see my connection." And trying like hell to put on a front during the day. *Put* on makeup. *Put* on a dress. *Get* out there. *Show* the world we're somebody. And then having to hide during the day and throw up somewhere and go somewhere and jam some coke up my nose. Get a drink at lunchtime just so I can make it until five o'clock. And then when it's five o'clock haul my ass over to the dealer's.

And I thought I was fine. You know? Somehow I really thought I was fine. When someone would confront me,

I would say "I'm fine. I'm really happy for you that you got cleaned up. That's nice you have a little club called AA. That's great but that ain't for me. I'm not that bad. I don't have that problem."

I started calling for help two years before I got clean and sober. I didn't know what I was calling for. I was just calling to help me come down. "Just please help me come down." Seven, eight in the morning, "Oh, God. Please help me come down."

And I'd be writing, "Please help me. Please help me. Please help me." All over paper, all over the place. It would be rolled up in balls all over the floor. "Please help me. Please help me. Please help me."

What am I supposed to do? *I don't know* what I'm supposed to do. *I'm fucking crazy.* And I don't know what it is. For *two* years this is what's goin' on. Wads of paper on the floor. "Please help me. Please help me."

And isolating from people and hiding bottles in the house and I said I would *never* do that. I would hide bottles and I would try to drink socially in front of people and I couldn't wait until they were gone so I could finish off some real booze.

And booze was *never* an issue. I didn't think I had any kind of booze problem at all. I kept the bottles in the house 'cause it was the social thing to do. There were so many excuses it was ridiculous. I was not an alcoholic. I *knew* I wasn't an alcoholic. My gramma was an alcoholic. My friends who were dead were alcoholics. I wasn't an alcoholic. I abused a little drugs here and there and I drank with it once in a while but I wasn't an *alcoholic*. Alcoholic was somebody who lived on the avenue and slept in the doorway and peed their pants. Forget the times I peed my pants in *public*. I'd just go home and clean up and pretend it never happened.

By this time I had tried to commit suicide a couple of times by deliberately overdosing. I'd played Russian roulette with myself — literally. I'd sit on the bed and load a .38 and put the bullets in the chamber and then I'd spin it around and then empty the bullets and then I'd stick one in it. And then I'd turn it around and then I'd take it to my head and I'd pull the trigger. And then when it wouldn't go off, I'd look at it and then I'd just burst out into these sweats really bad. Because for a semi-sane instant I would realize what I had just did.

I lost four jobs in one month, I just couldn't hang onto any work. But this one job, I wanted it so bad 'cause I just knew I could do it. I knew I could be somebody. It was this paralegal job and I knew I could do it. I knew it. I knew it. I knew it.

I missed the interview 'cause I overdosed on hallucinogenics and ended up in the hospital. But I got the job. They had lots of medical leave time and I used it up as fast as I got it 'cause I would be so hung over.

I represented people in administrative hearings on public assistance issues and one day I won a hearing. I'd won hearings before and this particular one was really important to me and I *won* the case. I was thrilled.

I'd been gone two weeks without really using anything and I was feeling like I've been so good I ought to get myself a little dope, you know. So I got just half a gram from this one dealer and I got off in the bathroom. Somehow part of me knew that half a gram wouldn't be enough but I had my kid with me and I think, "How about if I just drop my kid off somewhere and I'll go get another half a gram?" I don't even remember what I did with my kid that night. I really honest-to-God don't remember.

So I went and got another half a gram. Well, that half a gram wasn't gonna get me anywhere and so I went and got a gram. And then I got a case of beer and I went back to the house and got everything I had that was worth anything. I'd already spent the rent money. I'd already spent everything in the little piggy bank. And I went to another dealer's house. And I was making liquor store runs all night long 'cause I was going through the booze really fast.

About five in the morning when the bars were closed I went to the store to get some pop and I look up in that curved mirror up in the store and I saw *me* — pale, with extremely dark circles under my eyes. My eyes were bloodshot. One was going off in another direction. I couldn't get them to line up. My nose was almost bleeding it was so red. My mouth was all dried out. My lips were all puffed up. And I thought, "*Jesus*, that's me!"

I went back to the dealers and I finished off some more dope but I was getting sick and I was crawling around the bathroom and I was shaking really bad and I was starting to hallucinate. I was throwin' up and I hadn't eaten since noon and now it's like six the next morning and I can't function. My mind is goin' nuts and I wish to God it would stop and I know I don't wanna come down. I'm scared to *death* to come down. But I know it's gonna happen. The dope is gonna run out. And I'm goin', "Please gimme some more dope. Please gimme some more dope. I'll do *anything* for you if you gimme some more dope."

And so I did anything for them so I could get some more dope. And then I left and went home. I tried to finish off the dope and I was tryin' to write at the same time 'cause I was afraid I was gonna die. I could feel death coming on and I tried to write. I thought, "Okay this is a letter to the Creator 'cause I don't know where else to go. I gotta write to You because I'm gonna die."

The pain was so bad in my chest, like a heart attack kind of pain. It was like these tight bands around my chest and sweat was running off of me. There was only two beers left and I was down to two lines of coke and it was scaring me to death and, "What am I gonna *do*?"

I had the TV on, I had the stereo on, I had everything on. I needed company. And an ad came on the TV about cocaine. I'm sittin' there choppin' up cocaine and drinkin' beer like crazy. I grabbed the telephone and I called the crisis line. I just start crying, "I'm an addict. I know I'm an addict." I fell on the floor and I'm not sure what happened then. I don't know how anybody got there. But I remember I went to my first meeting at noon that day. Shaking really bad. Coming down really bad. And wanting help, I mean really wanting help. Not just writing onto pieces of paper.

I was clean for fifty-two days and it was *horrible*. It was lots of hallucinations and DTs. I couldn't hang on and I lost it. I went back out and I got really shitfaced and I couldn't stop crying about the deaths of my friends and all the stuff that happened.

I got drunk to the vomiting, blackout stage and I was crammin' coke up my nose. I was free-basin'. I was just doin' this as fast as I could and still goin' to meetings. Until somebody came up to me and said, "You look like hell," threw a quarter in my face and told me to call the treatment centre. So I did.

They said I could be admitted in three days. Well I stayed loaded as much as I could, but I didn't make it till the third day. I overdosed again and my sponsor and the guy I was goin' out with at the time, who is now my husband, took me to the treatment centre that night and admitted me into detox.

I hated everybody in the program. I would literally drag counsellors down the hall to look at the *rat* problem they had in that treatment centre. And I would be *pissed off* at them because they had spiders all over their tables and nobody would look. I would be so mad. I didn't realize how bad my DTs were. I really didn't. Boy, was it a surprise to wake up and see how near death I was. And all that denial. Incredible, incredible amounts of denial. My hallucinations were not completely gone until a year after being in the program.

I didn't know I had blackouts. I didn't know what they were. I just thought you woke up a few days later. I didn't know that's what people called them so when they asked me if I had blackouts I said, "No, what are those?" It took a sponsor in AA to tell me what they were and I sure as hell had 'em. (*laughs*) I felt so embarrassed.

I got my treatment paid for by the company I worked for, so I was damn lucky there. And they supported me at work too. When I went back to work I would be given time to go to meetings at lunchtime 'cause I needed it. I really feel grateful to them for that.

It was not an easy trip for me to get clean and sober. A year after I had been in the program, I spent five weeks in a mental hospital. It didn't make me feel real proud but I mentally couldn't handle anything. I had to do massive amounts of sexual abuse therapy. I'm still in therapy. I still have times of rage. But it's better. It's not as bad as it used to be. It was a big accomplishment after a year and a half in the program when I could say, "I'm Diane. I'm an addict-alcoholic and I've gone six weeks without physically abusing myself." Or, "I've gone two months now without thinking about suicide." Took a long time and it's still work. Sobriety is a constant effort. I'm one drink and one drug away from being back into it full-bore.

In a lot of ways I feel that I've been to the edge and back. I've really been to the edge mentally. I mean I was *gone*. I've definitely been a looney bin candidate a number of times. Part of my sobriety is acknowledging that as long as I'm making progress I don't have to be perfect. I always wanted to compare myself to perfection and I don't need to do that today.

I'll tell you one thing. I am *utterly* grateful for my sobriety and for every person who has had any impact on me at all with sobriety, whether I hated them or not. Because it took all of that stuff to get me to this point where I can even talk about it.

I know, and enough doctors told me this, that if I had continued even one more day I would have been dead. I just couldn't stop. I'd been on coke for ten years. I shot it. I free-based it. I smoked it till my nose hemorrhaged. I'm talkin' real hemorrhage (*laughs*) where they medevac you out.

Yeah, alcohol took me to strange new places. And I thought I'd seen it all when I was a kid. The fighting and so much blood. My therapist says I suffer from post-traumatic stress disorder. I thought that was only for war victims or something.

All I know is that I get excited when I think about *givin'* some of my sobriety to another person. It's like that's the best thing. It makes me happy if I can reach somebody else or help somebody else know that they're not alone. Nothin' motivates me more than seein' somebody who's in that position and see a *little* spark happenin' because I shared some of myself with them.

When people want to share some of their stories and, "Oh God, I've never told anybody this," I feel like, "I doubt you're gonna tell me something that I haven't already done. I *really* doubt it. I mean, it's *possible,* but there ain't a whole lot I haven't done myself. I've been there."

I don't care what somebody has done in their drug and alcohol usage. If they can get sober and share something, that's all that matters.

The journey in sobriety has not been easy for me. But I feel like the dark clouds are gone. The self-loathing is gone. The hate is gone. I don't know if there's a happy ending. There's *hope*. For the first time I believe there's hope. I do have mixed feelings. I still have depression, it's just not as deep. And I still have sadness over losses.

It's in recent years, being clean and sober, that I thought, "When I take care of myself, I take care of a member of the tribe."

And that was quite a thought, you know. I'm helpin' to take care of the tribe when I don't drink and use. And that's an important thought for me. It's been real hard for me to do things just for myself. It helps me when I think, "I'm a member of the tribe and I'm taking care of this percentage of this tribe when I take care of me."

7

DRUGS

*"I was up to thirty or forty hits a day . . . I used to crank
more and more drugs into my veins to see how high or
how stoned I could get."*

Compared to alcoholism, drug abuse is a relatively recent
phenomenon in native communities. Nevertheless, it is a
serious problem and no native community is too remote
to have a "drug problem."

In some ways, drug use is more complex than alcoholism, since it involves three distinct segments of the
native population and three broad categories: illegal street
drugs, solvents and prescription drugs.

Used by teenagers and young adults, street drugs
(everything from marijuana, hashish and LSD to speed,
heroin and cocaine) can be found in every native community, no matter how small or remote.

Solvents are primarily used by native children and
teenagers who are either not old enough or not affluent
enough to buy alcohol or street drugs. These young people are the "sniffers" who inhale everything from felt-tip
markers and cooking spray to airplane glue and gasoline.

129

The third category involves highly addictive prescription drugs: sedatives, painkillers and diet pills. The people who get hooked on this type of drug are usually grown-ups, particularly women. They become addicted unintentionally and unwittingly as a by-product of medical treatment. Once addicted, though, they feed their drug habits with the help of irresponsible doctors and a thriving black market.

The extent of native drug use was measured in a 1984 survey by the Federation of Saskatchewan Indian Nations. The survey found that nearly half the Indian adults surveyed (47 percent) said they had used drugs in the previous year. The survey also said that 21 percent of the nine hundred people questioned had a drug problem, mostly with illegal street drugs.

MARINE is the fifty-two-year-old Stoney grandmother in Chapter 1 whose great-grandfather sold the family's last horse for a barrel of whiskey.

My husband took sick and he had an operation. I thought he was going to get well but the doctor told me that he wasn't gonna live long. I asked him how long. He said he was gonna die, the longest would be three months. I started to cry and I got upset. He prescribed me some pills — tranquillizers and sleeping pills — which I took.

I was drinking too, off and on. I kept on taking them and never realized that I got addicted to them. The pills were easier to get than the alcohol and the effects were more dangerous too 'cause you got so silly and so stupid. Like you seem to know what you're doing but yet people will see you acting so crazy.

Like this one time, me and my daughters were going Christmas shopping. This daughter and me were going in one vehicle and the other two were going in the truck. I was going to cash a cheque and when we got to the bank I got out and they left. I thought we were gonna follow them but instead my daughter just came back home. I asked her, "Aren't we going to Calgary too?"

She said, "No. We're going home. We can go another time."

All this time I thought I was okay and I wasn't. A couple days later she told me that all the time we were going there I was pretending to eat and when we got to the bank, she said I asked, "Where's my hot dog?"

I thought I was eating a hot dog. (*laughs*) And I thought I knew what I was doing! So damn crazy. When they came back, my other daughters, they asked me, "What did you have on your way back home? A hamburger?"

JEFF is thirty years old. He's from the Stl'atl'imx Nation in the southern mountains of British Columbia. He grew up in a Vancouver suburb and has been sober for six months.

When I drank I used a number of different drugs. I smoked marijuana. I smoked hash. I tried hallucinogenic drugs, LSD, and I'd tried cocaine. On one occasion, during a wake for a biker friend, a number of us had started snorting a white powder. I was half in the bag at the time and I felt that, "Jeez, a white powder. Must be cocaine."

So I just went right at it and started getting as much up my nose as I could. And the next morning I woke up and I was in a cold sweat and the bed was drenched. My friend Tom said I looked like a bag of shit and asked me how I was doin'. And I said, "I'm not feeling too hot. That had to be the worst coke I ever had in my whole life."

And he said, (*laughs*) "That wasn't coke. That was junk."

We had been snorting heroin all night! At that time I realized I had no idea whatsoever what I was doin' to myself. I'd no regard for what I was puttin' into my body, let alone any respect for my body.

That same day, which was a Sunday, we decided to jump into Jerry's Volkswagen and drive to the U.S. and proceeded to put away the better part of a twenty-four-pack of Boone's Farm Apple Wine. I didn't even like wine, and this stuff tasted like syrup. But it sure did the trick. After about three bottles, I started to feel a lot better.

JOSIE, thirty-one years old, is of Aztec ancestry from Los Angeles. Short and perky with flashing brown eyes, she has been sober for eleven years.

Paint sniffing. How could I forget that? That's something I did, oh gosh, almost two years. I started doing that stuff at fourteen years old. There was these girls I used to hang around with and that was something they had always done. I finally decided to try it and I liked it. It was a cheap high. A can of paint you can buy for less than two dollars.

The only colours we would sniff were silver, bright copper enamel or brass. But the brass would dry up too fast. There was a big difference between copper and other colours. It tasted better, okay?

When I first started, I was sniffing from a sock. On the foot of the sock you would spray it till it was soaked and then you'd roll it up like you were putting away laundry and just stick it in your mouth. We didn't sniff it through our nose, we sniffed it through our mouth. But that was something you had to keep on doing to keep high. You had to keep that thing in your mouth. If not, you wouldn't stay high. It would last maybe five, ten minutes. That stuff, I really liked it. (*laughs*)

And I used to sniff out of a bread bag. That was probably one of the clumsiest things to do because after a while the bag would just dissolve and I used to look like I was dipped in paint. So when I would get spotted with paint, after the paint would dry, I would get a razor and scrape it off.

I knew a couple people who just became total vegetables from the paint. This one guy that I knew, he couldn't even talk. There was a lot of people that would sniff just about anything. I could never do that. I had some pretty bad trips with paint, really scary, because once in a while I would smoke and I felt like I was going to explode, you know, my head. I would feel this rumbling sound and it was just a weird trip.

I noticed how addicted I was getting on paint. I was getting these really sharp pains on the top of my head and then when I would do paint again they would go away.

When I got into high school, I got a job working in an office but I felt that people could smell it. Anyway, when I got this job, I just decided to cold-turkey it. It was really getting to me, getting to my head, the smell. I felt that no matter how clean I was, that odour was there. It didn't matter how many times I brushed my teeth or how many sticks of gum I chewed, there was always this awful taste in my mouth. I could feel these fumes in my head and you could see this stuff, the fumes, coming out of my mouth. It was really starting to gross me out.

❧

GORDON'S STORY

Gordon is a beefy, fast-talking thirty-nine-year-old Ojibway with a hearty laugh. He grew up in the Cabbagetown section of Toronto and is now an estimator for a steel company. Gordon was interviewed in his Toronto apartment. He has been sober for six years.

When we were fourteen or fifteen years of age, we used to spend most of our time up in Riverdale Park. There was about four or five of us that used to hang out there all the time. We'd go find the rubbies or the old alkies standing around the corners. We used to go up to one of them and say, "Go buy two bottles of wine. Get yourself one and buy us one."

I remember the night I first drank. I got so loaded the guys had to carry me. I was shitting and pissing all the way home. My brother tried to straighten me up when I got home. He did the best he could but my mother still saw that I was bombed when she got home. I got grounded for the first time in my life.

But it was great. That first drink made me just as good as anyone I was with, just the sense that at one point in my life I *belonged*. It just made everything ease inside. It was just like taking a massive dose of Valium (*laughs*) and everything just settled out really nice.

I turned to drugs because I was under age and it was difficult to get alcohol and I was tired of getting grounded by my mother every time I came home drunk. With drugs she couldn't tell, so I stopped the alcohol and moved into drugs.

I got married at eighteen and for three years I didn't

drink or do drugs. That marriage broke up and I got into drugs again. I started dealing and within a year I was mainlining —speed, MDA — it gets the heart going. I was up to thirty or forty hits a day. My arms were black and blue, up and down.

I did that for two years. Many overdoses. I lived right across the street from Wellesley Hospital and any time I had an O.D. all's I had to do was go down the elevator, cross the street and into emergency. They'd shoot me down. I'd walk back over and go back upstairs and start over again. That's the insanity of it.

I was really out on a death wish. I used to crank more and more drugs into my veins to see how high or how stoned I could get. I kept doing more and more to find out what my limit was. I come close to it many, many times and somehow I was always saved.

I almost died once in the Wellesley Hospital. I remember going in and my heart was just going like crazy. Some doctor started listening to my heart and couldn't believe what he was hearing. He brought one of those little EKG machines over, hooks it up, turns it on and the old needle was going so fast he couldn't believe it. The paper was shooting out and he says, "This has got to be wrong."

And he grabs another machine, hooks it up and it's doing the same thing. And he couldn't believe it. (*laughs*) Then he called for the electronic one, with the beeps that go across? Well, he turned that one on and the beeps were going across that machine so quickly that next you know I'm surrounded by four or five doctors all of them sticking needles into me all over the place and then they tried to shoot me down, which was an interesting experience because they were worried they were going to stop my heart. So here's the doctor shooting the Valium up and here's another doctor standing there with those electric paddles just in case they stopped the heart. Well, they never did. (*laughs*) Thank God.

I was dealing drugs, got busted and did time. I got out and turned to alcohol to get off the drugs. My intake of alcohol became greater. I was still popping the odd pill here and there. I was a weekend junkie.

Eventually I hit the bottom of my drinking. What happened is that alcohol and drugs no longer made living liveable. I no longer felt good when I drank, no matter how much I drank. It was bringing me down. I was sitting around crying and I couldn't understand why. I just wanted to die and that was it.

I used to get Tylenol IIs from the doctor, so one night I just had enough and I walked over to the kitchen sink and just picked up all the pills and downed about fifty of them. I was already half in the bag drunk. I just wanted to die. That was April 27, 1984.

I was staring at the kitchen wall and I guess the will to live just all of a sudden kicked in and I asked myself, "What are you doing?"

I picked up the phone and phoned my brother. This was two o'clock in the morning. So my brother came over and he got me up to the hospital. Some doctor gave me something to bring up all these pills and I was violently sick. Later, when there was nobody around to watch the halls, I got dressed and went back home.

Unfortunately, I gave them the right address where I lived and a half-hour later the police were there and they arrested me under the Canada Mental Health Act. They politely took me back and put me up on the tenth floor of the hospital, which is the psychiatric part. I was up there for a week and they eventually let me out. After I left the hospital I went to AA. That's been six and a half years now.

The only reason I went to AA was to get my wife and daughter back. I had no desire to quit drinking. I thought I would be able to drink again one day as a social drinker and every time I went to AA they were telling me I'm never going to drink again. I don't wanna hear that.

So my motives for stopping drinking were totally wrong. It took me a year and a half in AA where I wanted to stop drinking.

I figured I was over the major hurdle when I accepted the fact that I've got this problem with alcohol. (*laughs*) Then it got worse. For the next thirteen months I literally thought I was going insane. Then I guess I hit another bottom, the emotional one, of the anger that was always building up and being released here, there and everywhere. In the second year of AA, the anger was starting to get worse.

My state of thinking was still really, really screwed up. They call it the merry-go-round. I couldn't keep any thought pattern going on any one issue. A thought would come in — it would go out. And another one would come in — go out. It was just a whole mesh of different thoughts and I couldn't make heads or tails out of anything. That went on for almost two and a half years.

I was at a point in my sobriety where I was getting ready to give up. Until January 18, 1987. It was a Sunday night. I remember sitting and thinking to myself, "Gord, you've been sober two and a half years now and you've still got as much anger now as you had when you walked in those doors. You haven't forgiven anybody. You're still mad at everybody. You're still mad at the world."

I was living with my niece at that time. I remember going home. I walked into my bedroom and something strange happened. I stopped and I could feel someone behind me. I turned and there was nothing there but then all of a sudden there was this tremendous warmth all around me. It felt very nice and very comforting. I felt there was something else there in that room and yet I was the only one standing in that room. And this was in the middle of winter and all of a sudden it was warm all around me. I describe it as being touched by the hand of God.

And then all of a sudden, the mind that kept spinning around, stopped and I was able to think. I was able to read that "12 and 12" (The Twelve Steps and Twelve Traditions of Alcoholics Anonymous) for the first time in two and a half years and understand it perfectly. I started reading and everything just made perfect sense. I thought, "How did I ever miss all this?" I've been reading it for two and a half years!

It was one of the best feelings I ever felt in my life. I've never felt anything like it before. It was like my mind totally emptied out of all the negativity and bad experiences. It was as if it was a bad dream and it was okay now. It was like I was given another chance to do something with my life. That night I had one of the best sleeps of my life.

I never used to read books. I could never sit down and read a book. But the next day I sat down and I was reading all these books. I read the Bible. I read other books giving myself positive thoughts instead of the negative thoughts that were there.

And I never had to look back. I never craved drink after that. Today I have the freedom of choice whether to drink or not. Up to that point of time, I still didn't have the control, the drink still had me. People look at you kind of weird when you talk about something like that.

AA is really my lifesaver. Without it I really don't think I would have recovered. Sitting within AA I used to think those people were keeping secrets from me because they weren't telling me how to be happy anymore because I was miserable. But I found their secret. They were telling me every time I went to a meeting. My problem is I didn't want to hear it. (*laughs*) Until one day I did. One day that little secret just turned on the old light bulb. The secret to the whole program is "have a belief." Have a belief in God or what you believe to be God.

For anyone who's trying to recover from alcoholism, don't give up. No matter how hard it gets, it will get worse before it gets better. As long as you don't give up, you will recover. (*laughs*)

8

IMAGES

"He started cracking a joke about a drunken squaw and he thought I was just gonna sit there and take it."

To most television viewers, a beer commercial is either an entertaining diversion or an annoying interruption that offers a chance to go to the kitchen or the bathroom. But to some people, the sight of white, frothy foam pouring over the side of a frosty glass filled with clear golden beer is a very powerful image. In fact, it is strong enough to drive some people to drink and it is strong enough to trigger angry reactions in many native people.

Many native people are also deeply affected by another powerful image — the linkage of native people and alcohol in the "drunken Indian" stereotype. One of the questions I asked people during the interviews for this book was: "What do you think when you hear non-native people say, 'All native people are drunks'?" Most native people said in response that they were outraged, but a surprising number of people agreed with it. However, the individual responses were not as important as the fact that *everyone* seems to have heard the remark at some time in their life. The stereotype of the "drunken Indian" is still alive and well.

If there is a stereotype involving the "sober Indian," it may be that sober people (like fat people) are happy and jolly. Obviously, that's not always the case because alcohol often scars and cripples the innocent.

HAL is a sixty-five-year-old Tsimshian and a retired air traffic controller. He is self-assured and confident, with a broad smile and a rich radio announcer's voice. Hal was interviewed in his home, a small bungalow in Anchorage, Alaska. He has been sober for seven years.

Society says, "All natives are drunks." Well, maybe so, because it does appear that "quote-quote" all natives are drunks. It's a tough statement and some people would resent hearing that or reading that. There's a lot of resentment among the native people towards the non-natives.

And some white people feel guilty about the treatment of the natives and they kind of go on a guilt trip, taking the blame for what's happening to the native people. I says, "Unh-unh." I says, "Who's responsible? We are."

Some of the white people might be responsible, true. But take a look at what the non-natives in general have brought to the country — sciences, invention, knowledge, the use of the mind, teaching, improving, providing for tomorrow. It is not the fault of the "quote-quote" white man that we are overpowered with technology. They sure most certainly did not force alcohol down our throats. It might appear that they did. But they did not.

We brought it on ourselves through ignorance or by choice, by failing to be adequately educated, to get the job skills and careers that are available. All of a sudden we find ourselves in a technological world and we don't have the educational skills, the job skills, the coping-with-life skills. In other words, we were unprepared for the changes.

Alcohol is a destroyer of our people. So long as it's in a bottle, it's harmless. But we pick up that bottle of our own volition. Nobody forces us to, so we self-destruct. It should be treated with the utmost respect and fear. Respect it like poisonous snakes or nitroglycerine or dynamite or gasoline. Just leave it the heck alone and respect it, not hate it.

MARGARET is a twenty-five-year-old Mohawk and calls herself a social drinker. She works as a youth counsellor and was interviewed in her office.

The beer commercials on TV really annoy me because the message they give is that all people that are popular are the people that drink. They don't show the persons that are drunk or falling off their chairs or young, pretty girls being hit on by slimy, greasy, ugly, gross-looking guys.

All the commercials are like that. They all show young people having a good time and being dressed up. All of them. They're all around the swimming pools. They don't show anybody with liver disease or kidney failure or anything like that in the hospital, you know. It just gives the impression that there are no consequences to drinking.

SERENA is a petite nineteen-year-old Alberta Cree with long black hair and a sparkling smile. A single parent, she has undergone treatment for alcoholism twice. She has been sober for five weeks.

I think, "How sick," you know? I don't wanna see this. Like even though this is TV, it's not my life anymore. To see commercials like that, it's like you can smell the awful smell of it. I want to get sick. It doesn't make me thirsty.

I get scared when I see those commercials because old memories, like little flashbacks come back. Like my father and my mother drinking. The fighting. The grandparents fighting. Seeing my uncles and aunties flip out when they're drunk. People look like they're having a good time and then by the end of the night everybody's scrapping, you know. Fights going on, somebody pulling a knife out. Shit like that.

Like all these different things, all these bad experiences, come to my head when I see those commercials.

BRODY, a twenty-nine-year-old Haida, was a binge drinker before entering a native treatment centre for alcoholism.

I don't like the idea of advertising at all. I think they should put warning labels on bottles like they do cigarettes. "Excessive drinking may cause death."

*DAVE is a soft-spoken thirty-one-year-old Chipewyan student.
His thick glasses and unimposing physique disguise his three
years of martial arts training. He drinks just one or two beers a
year.*

I remember once hearing it, that "all natives are drunks,"
in a bar in Drayton Valley, Alberta, two years ago. This guy
was sitting at the same table with us and he was talking
to a whole bunch of his white friends, trying to be Mr.
Fucking Joe Cool and he started cracking a joke about a
drunken squaw and he thought I was just gonna sit there
and take it. He thought I wasn't gonna say anything. He
thought I was just another wimpy little Indian who was
gonna let him get away with this because the bar was full
of white people.

And my first thought was, "Oh, you mean white men
don't get drunk?"

And my second thought was, "How can you be so ignorant? Not every Indian is a drunk. I'm not a drunk."

And I remember my third reaction. I said, "You little
fucker." I kicked the table onto his lap and punched the
shit out of him. I beat him. I beat him real bad.

BELLA'S STORY

*Bella is a darkly serious thirty-one-year-old Cree from a
reserve in northern Manitoba. Although she has been a non-
drinker just about all her life, she has been deeply scarred by
alcoholism.*

I tried drinking just a couple of times when I was young,
but I couldn't hack it. There was five of us girlfriends.
The third time I told them, "I can't do this. I don't like

the taste of it. I don't like the smell of it. It's gross." I just left it alone after that.

My parents used to make a lot of homebrew when they were drinking. It used to make them crazy. I think that's why I decided to live a sober life. They were gone all the time. They used to come home only twice a month: welfare day and family allowance day. They were in Thompson all the time. That was from the time I was eight till I was nineteen. There was eleven of us. Five boys and six girls.

My one granny used to go and tell the welfare workers that we were alone. I was scared that they would take the kids. The social workers would come by and look all over the house.

"Where are the kids?"

I said, "Oh, they're outside playing somewhere."

"Where's your mum?"

"She's visiting. She went shopping."

I used to lie. Quite a bit. I never told them I thought they were drinking somewhere. To this day, I don't understand it myself, why I used to lie for them. And I continued lying for years. (*laughs*)

They got us one time. I didn't know they were coming. I was always at the door, guarding when my mum was gone, eh? But one time we slept in late and the next thing I knew she was pushing. She says, "Get up. You have to go."

And I said, "Where?"

She says, "To a foster home."

I said, "Why?"

And she says, "Because nobody's here. Your mum's not here."

So I said, "I can take care of them."

She said, "But you're under sixteen."

So she took us to some foster home. The kids were all sad. We were sitting there and I was making up this plan in my head, eh? So I told them, "Go play outside for a while. Just wait for me, I'll be out there. We'll run away."

So they did. I just sitting there pretending to watch TV and then I walked out. I said, "Okay! Come on, let's go!"

So we ran into the bush and we ran home. When we got there my mum was home and she was wondering where we were and I told her. When the welfare worker came back I told her, "See? There's my mum. She was home all this time." (*laughs*)

That's the only time they caught us. Those other times they could never do it 'cause I used to always hide the kids. I'd tell them to crawl under the house. Or else I'd shut them up in the attic. I'd hide them where it was dark. They're all scared of the dark now. Even the older ones.

I got to hate those social workers. And I used to hate the minister. He used to come over try to help me out. I didn't want no part of him either.

It was me who raised up all those kids. Nine of us. I've got one older brother ahead of me. But he was living with my grandmother. My brothers, my sisters, they still call me "Mum."

My mum gave away two of the kids but they came back after she quit drinking. Those two I don't really know. I'm not attached to them at all. I know they're my brother and sister, that's all I know.

I can remember the time they were given away. My mum gave them away when she was drunk at a party. This person would come and say, "Your mum gave me this kid," and she'd run off with this kid, this little baby.

The first one she gave away was a year, I think. And the next one she gave away was two months. And the third she was trying to give away was about three months.

That's the one I went and got back — once at three months, once at four months, once at five months. Three times she gave her away. Three times I went back and got her. At that time I was twelve. That one still calls me "Mum" all the time.

What makes me mad is my sister that was given away. She's twenty and just this year she told me in that home she was in, she was sexually abused by that stepfather. That makes me angry. I couldn't believe it when she was telling me. She was abused all the time — sexually, mentally. It bothers me. I kept wishing I could have gone and got her too.

I took good care of the kids, I think. (*laughs*) I managed. If my mum didn't come home on family allowance day, I'd forge her name and go cash it. I used to watch my mum how she wrote her name and then start practising. Other times I went to lie to the welfare office. I used to say, "Give me this thing, my mum's sick."

The other times I used to go work for somebody. Go wash dishes or clean house. I used to make five bucks, ten bucks. Then I'd go buy groceries.

We went to school too. I took all of them to school. When there was three younger ones that didn't go to school yet, I used to take them to my other granny's. My granny'd take care of them till after school, then I'd go pick them up again.

It was hard but I managed. I 'member my mum teaching me how to clean up a house when I was seven, how to wash clothes, standing on a chair, with one of those old washing machines where you put gas and you pull this cord. A big motor and it makes a loud noise. (*laughs*) And standing on a chair to cook on a wood stove. She taught me those things. Guess that was her plan to be leaving us all the time. That's what I thought of it after.

When I made the decision to live a sober life I was about twelve or thirteen. It was when my dad was beating up my mum. Me and my brother jumped my dad not to bother my mum. I said to myself, "I'm not going to do this. I'm not gonna get drunk when I grow up, when I have kids."

Alcohol had a lot of effect on my family. All of us are mean people. We grew up to be mean. The whole family is. They're just mean to everybody. A lot of anger.

They beat up their kids. I used to do that but I quit. (*laughs*) I started realizing that's not good. I used to go to Adult Children of Alcoholics. It helped me quite a bit, understanding what I went through, the anger I kept inside me for twenty-five years.

That's the other thing that really bugs me. I am angry that I didn't have a childhood. Especially when these southern people talk about, "What I did when I was a kid." The way they talk, it's so exciting, eh? What they did when they were kids.

I just sit there and I can't talk about anything I did when I was a child. All I can talk about is how I took care of these kids all the time.

9

QUITTING

"I didn't go to any treatment centre. I didn't quit through AA. I quit from hearing my own teachings."

The Haudenosaunee call alcohol "the mind-changer" but they could just as well have called it "the mind-eraser" for its ability to erase a person's short-term and long-term memory. Long-term drinkers get "on the wagon" (and fall off) many times before they are finally able to quit for good, but the details of these many failed attempts are usually lost in a blurry alcoholic fog.

Despite alcohol's obliterative qualities, though, most drinkers can vividly remember all the details of the last day they drank. Their transformation, from long-term drunkenness to sobriety, is often triggered by a single dramatic incident that sears the details into their brain and engraves the emotions of a near-religious experience onto their soul.

ROSEMARIE is a forty-nine-year-old Ojibway. She quit drinking seventeen years ago and lives in Toronto.

I tried to quit drinking on my own several times. I would go for six weeks, eight weeks, and go back drinking for two or three days and it would be a total disaster. I never went to a detox centre, but there was times that I was isolated in my apartment and was afraid to go out. One time, I was a couple of days off a drunk and I did call the detox centre and they said to me, "I'm sorry we don't take anybody unless they're drunk."

So I thought that was kind of a stupid thing and a good excuse for me to continue. I said, "Okay, I'll go out and buy a bottle and I'll call you back."

TINA is a forty-nine-year-old Stoney from southern Alberta. A tiny, quiet woman, she quit drinking fourteen years ago.

I was a mean drunk. I had a bad temper and I was mad at everybody. One night we were at our house and we had two other couples that were drinking with us and I must have filled the bathtub up with water. Course, I didn't know at the time I was doing this 'cause I was in a blackout. My husband was so drunk I just grabbed him and he couldn't even resist. He just followed me where I took him. I dumped him in there and was holding him under the water.

My cousin's wife wondered what I was doing, so she came to check and here I was holding him under the water. She grabbed my hands and moved me out of the washroom and by then my husband sort of sobered up and sat up and they unplugged the tub. And we just continued drinking again.

The next day he didn't remember anything about it and I didn't remember any of it. My cousin's wife told me what

I had done. That scared me, that I had come that close to killing another human being, so I thought I'd better do something about my drinking. I realized that if I continued drinking I could actually murder somebody. At that time there was a courtworker, Bob Ogle, who used to serve out here in the community. He used to try and get me to come to AA and I would always tell him I was not an alcoholic. I used to resent him but after I damn near drowned my husband in the bathtub I thought I better go to see him. I told him what I had almost done. At that time there were no treatment centres and he said, "Well, you get yourself to AA."

ELSTON is the eighteen-year-old Stoney who, as described in Chapter 6, resumed drinking after a vicious brawl with his brother that left the two of them with multiple injuries. Elston began drinking heavily when he was twelve years old. He was interviewed at Stoney Medicine Lodge and has a distinctive accent that makes him pronounce "alcohol" as "ackahol."

They didn't want me in the house 'cause I was drunk. So I grabbed a rock and I threw it through the window. And I grabbed another rock and I smashed the car window. Later on, I was on a hill with a twenty-six, slicing my wrists. I didn't know why. It was just ackahol taking over me. I passed out there. The next morning I woke up and walked down the hill and went in my house and told them, "What are you staring at me for?"

They told me, "We press charges against you. What the heck did you do?"

I told them I didn't know what I do. They told me that I break the window, smashed the car. I thought they were gonna lock me up if I go to court again 'cause that was my second time. I was scared, eh? My uncle came in and he told me, "Ackahol is taken control over you. You need to go to treatment." He was mad at me, uh? Whipping me and telling me to quit drinking.

I went to court and I told the judge that I need to go to treatment. He let me go. I was in treatment for three days and I thought, "This is not for me," and I just left.

My uncle got mad at me again and he told me, "If you don't want to quit drinking, come into the sweat lodge with me." He was mad at me.

I told him, "Okay." I couldn't say nothing, 'cause he was a medicine man and I went into the sweat lodge with my uncle and my auntie.

Sweat lodge — it's hot, eh? Spirit came in and I was burned. My skin was burned. My hair was just all dried up and I was just crying. They didn't burn though. I was the only one that burned. I was trying to get out but my auntie was in the door. When the sweat lodge was over I told my uncle, "How come you guys didn't burn and I was burned?"

He told me, "That's ackahol trying to get out. That bad spirit in you is trying to get out. The spirit that's making you do stupid things. Getting you into trouble."

So I went back home and I thinked about it. And I haven't drink for four months ever since that sweat lodge.

DONALD is a baby-faced twenty-four-year-old Alberta Metis with a lengthy criminal record. He took his last drink eight months ago, shortly before he was jailed for his latest offence. He later transferred from jail to a native treatment centre, where he was interviewed.

I done a lot of crazy stuff because of drinkin'. Takin' knives after friends. Other times I'd try to kill my friends by shootin' at them because I'd lost a fight. I had a lot of anger inside me, with my father drinkin' and me goin' in and out of foster homes ever since I was five years old. And bein' child abused and all that.

In 1976, I lost a brother. He was only seven years old. He was killed by a drunk driver in a semi. I was ten years old. This semi hit him and he died of brain damage. I was very upset because my brother was my best friend. He meant the world to me, and I was just really pissed off then.

I had a lot of hatred in my life. I didn't really care. I didn't give a shit about myself or others. My heavy drinkin' caused me to get in trouble with the law. I ended up doin' some time. I was assaulted by police officers and pushed around by guards. I was gettin' really tired of that. So I had a lot of negativeness inside me while I was servin' time.

I didn't really want to live anymore. So I tried to commit suicide in jail by tryin' to hang myself. But I was caught before I had the chance. Other times I tried to commit suicide at a halfway house by O.D.'ing. Didn't succeed. Ended up in the hospital. I felt depressed.

I was turnin' into a psycho because of drunk-ness. I was dangerous to myself, I was dangerous to other people. So one night after I got out, I decided to break the law on purpose and end up in jail and quit drinkin' this way. I knew there was Alcoholics Anonymous, but I didn't call them. Why, I don't really know. I guess I just didn't want to be a bother to anyone at that time.

I had decided what I was gonna do. I was gonna get drunk and really pissed and I was gonna break a window or somethin' like that. But I stole a Corvette and ended up in a high-speed chase on purpose for them to catch me. I was really suicidal at that time. I just didn't give a shit. I just wanted to get off the street. I felt if I was in jail, it was the only way I could quit drinkin'. So I put myself in jail because I didn't feel I could do it.

This happened February 2nd of this year. My time is up at the end of this month. After I had been involved with AA for some time in jail, I put a request to do the rest of my time at Poundmaker's. Poundmaker's Lodge was willin' to take me to do my last few days here. The only reason why they were takin' me was I was askin' for help and I wanted to get some treatment. I know for a fact if I stick with AA, I can do it this time. I've been sober for eight months now. (*laughs*) I sobered up the hard way.

CARDINAL is a twenty-seven-year-old Saskatchewan Cree with a broad smile and an open, easygoing manner. He wears pearl-button shirts, blue jeans, cowboy boots and a cowboy hat. He began drinking heavily in his early teens and has been sober for seven years. He's now an addictions counsellor in a native treatment centre.

When I was younger I was really shy and I never could go to a function or do things that the other guys did — like ask girls out or ask them if they wanted to dance. I just didn't have the courage to do that. But I found out that after I had a few drinks I was John Travolta. I'd ask anybody out and do just about anything.

I never saw anything wrong with my drinking. I just never thought about it. Everybody drank and it was no big deal. Everybody got drunk. Everybody blacked out.

Everybody did crazy things when they were drinking. It was normal from where I come from. So I didn't ever feel I was out of the ordinary. I thought I was normal.

From the first time I drank I blacked out, so I don't know what it's like to drink sociably. I remember one time coming out of a blackout, opening my eyes and having my father below me and I was beating the shit out of him. I don't know why I did it. I don't know what happened. I just came to and I was on top of my father and I was beating the shit out of him. His nose was all bloody and stuff and I freaked out and I took off and I don't think I came back for about a month.

Another time I woke up and I walked into the room and I was wondering why my dad wouldn't look at me. I was wondering why he wouldn't talk to me. I told my mum, "What's wrong with Dad?"

And she just blasted me. She told me to get out. I didn't understand why. I just woke up and thought everything was fine. And then I looked at my dad and his face was all puffy one side. He was all beat up. I guess I had punched him out the night before. That's why he wouldn't talk to me and that's why he was avoiding me.

I've done some pretty crazy things — breaking into people's houses and a lot of vandalism when I was younger. Flattening some dude's tires — that can be repaired, but I had hurt severely somebody that I love very much. Those are probably the two worse things I've ever done.

The way I started to sober up was this. I was living in Calgary and I had gotten paid a lot of money and I went on a drunk with my cousins for about a week. After all my money was gone, we were in this van passing through the Sarcee reserve. They asked me if I had any more money and I looked in my pockets and I said, "No."

And they said, "Do you have any more in the bank?" and I said, "No."

So they stopped, opened up the side door and threw me out. Holy shit! I couldn't believe it. These are my cousins, eh?

So I picked myself up off the gravel and started walking, swearing, cursing, you name it. I was hung over. It was pouring rain, too. It was a lousy day, (*laughs loudly*) but it was the turning point in my life.

It was funny, you know, it occurred to me that the road I was walking down was called "The Last Stretch." It's a road leading to the graveyards. It's the last road that you take, your last ride on the reserve. So I was walking down that road and I was thinking, "Jeez, of all the places to get dropped off, they dropped me off on this road. There must be two hundred roads on the reserve and they threw me off on this one."

Up to this point I had been thinking about quitting because of the shit I was getting into and I thought, "Jeez, I gotta quit." I felt that I was on my last stretch, something told me it was one way or the other and I didn't want to go down that road. I was only twenty years old, man. I was scared. I was lonely. I was pissed off. I was hung over and I just decided to do something about it.

A friend of mine who had quit drinking lived down that road so I went to see him and he took me to a treatment centre on the reserve. They took me to a detox centre in Calgary. I was in detox for seven days.

One of my counsellors was a coloured fella, big guy, a body builder. He says, "Your name's Cardinal, right?"

And I said, "Yep."

And he says, "I'm your counsellor. I'm so-and-so."

And I said, "Yeah, yeah, yeah."

He says, "So you wanna sober up, do ya?"

I said, "Yes sir."

He says, "Well, what are you willing to give up?"

I said, "What are you talking about?"

He says, "What are you willing to sacrifice to stay sober?"

And I tol' him, "Nothing."

And he says, "Well, you might as well leave now."

And I thought, "This guy's being a real jerk."

And he says, "You're going to have to sacrifice some stuff. You can't live the way you used to live. You're gonna have to get rid of the friends. You gotta get rid of the old lifestyle. You can't hang out some of the places you used to. That's what I'm talking about. Are you willing to sacrifice some of those?"

And I told him, "Boy, you're an asshole. You hardly even know me and now you're telling me how to live my life. You're trying to tell me who I can hang out with and who I can't. You don't know anything about my friends. So how can you sit there and tell me what I have to do to stay sober? And you're telling me to get rid of all my buddies?"

He says, "Are they real buddies?"

And I said, "Yes, they are. I grew up with these boys. I partied with them. I chased girls with them. I went to school with them. They're not friends, they're like family. And you're telling me I have to give these guys up?"

He says, "Do they drink?"

And I said, "Yep."

He says, "Okay. Wait here, I'll be right back." He came back and he had a clipboard. He says, "When did you come in?"

And I said, "About a week ago."

He says, "Did you come in the same time as Wendy, John, Bill and so on?"

And I said, "Yes."

And he says, "Here, check this out."

And he spun his clipboard and showed me this chart. He says, "Take a look at that, Cardinal. Everybody else in this goddam place has had a visitor except for you. Where in the hell's all your friends?"

And I could have choked the son of a bitch, but he was huge. I said, "Well, they didn't know I was coming here."

He says, "Here's two bucks. Pay phone's outside. Phone 'em."

I thought, "What an asshole."

I grabbed the two bucks, changed it, and I went and I phoned a bunch of buddies. And, no kidding, my heart was breaking while I was on the phone because every last one of them, I was tellin' 'em, "I'm in detox, man. Can you come visit me?"

And they came up with a million excuses why they wouldn't come and visit me. I can't remember all of them but they were pretty good at the time. None of them would come visit me.

And the counsellor says, "Well, when they comin'?"

I had a couple of quarters left. I threw them back at 'im and I said, "They're not."

I was pissed off because he had made his point.

He says, "Well, I bet if I gave you some more quarters and I bought you a hotel room across the street, gave you a good bag of pot and a couple cases of beer and then you phoned, think they'd come and visit you then?"

And I thought, "Yeah, I betcha they would."

He said, "You're such a sucker, Cardinal. They're not comin' to visit you. When you gonna figure out? When the pot's gone, when the booze is gone, when the money's gone — they're gone." And then he left the room.

That slammed me up against the wall. It snapped me out of it. That helped me.

From the detox I went to a treatment centre. From that centre I went to another centre to another centre to another centre. Right in a row. And by the time I got out of all these treatment centres, I was nine months sober. That's how I quit.

LIZ is a fifty-eight-year-old Odawa who grew up on a reserve in central Ontario. She drank heavily for thirty years before she quit drinking in 1975. She is now an addictions counsellor.

I hated being an Indian. I wanted to be white and I didn't want to be Indian because of the put-down we had from white people. I even dyed my hair red. I even married a white man so not to be Indian. I never wanted to associate with Indian people when I was drinking. It was always with white people that I drank wit'. I hated being Indian. I've always said I'd never marry a man who would beat me up like my father beat my mother. That is one of the reasons why I married a white man.

When I was drinking I was a real heavy drinker. I've been arrested for drunkenness quite a few times because I was always with the bootleggers when they were being raided. I guess I got arrested about seven or eight times.

When I was drinking I took a knife to my husband. But he ran out the door and he called the police. I t'ought it was him at the door. I opened the door and I went after the police with the knife. I got arrested. I was handcuffed, put in jail.

They put me in a psychiatric hospital in North Bay and from that time on I was in and out of there for two years. Every time I would come out I would slash my wrists just to get back in there. I never meant to kill myself, it wouldn't be deep cuts, just enough to get me back into the hospital where I t'ought I was safe, where I didn't have to worry about anything.

I tried to quit drinking quite a few times. One time I quit for thirty days. That was in the sixties when my mother died and her last words to me was, "Liz, quit yer drinking and start lookin' after your daughter." That was her last words to me. I said I would. But I never quit. I just quit that one month for her. After she died I could hardly wait for thirty days to be over, then I went on a big drunk.

In the last month of my drinking days I was really climbing walls because I was going through a forty-ouncer of scotch a day. Plus that wasn't enough. I was into LSD, hash and grass. I had a really rough time.

The worst hangover I ever had was when I had been drinking for about three weeks nonstop. I was home alone and I felt someone laying beside me and I didn't know who it was and there was an awful smell. I never smelled anything like that before. Only at a funeral, like in the summer how the body starts to smell — that's the way it smelled. And I got really scared. I couldn't move. I couldn't yell. That was one of the scariest feelings I ever had and I never drank for two weeks after that.

But then I got lonely and I went drinking again. I was going through DTs, so I went over to my brother's who had been sober for five years. I told him I was having such a hard time. I slept in the spare bedroom but I left the lights on. Even with the lights on, this man came in the room. I've always been terrified of bats and he had bats. He was throwing bats at me and I screamed, so my brother sat with me all night, trying to talk to me about what alcohol does. But still I couldn't quit. I couldn't leave the alcohol alone.

I tried AA and it didn't work for me. I even went to medicine people. Still it didn't work. Finally my sister and her husband were on their way to Wisconsin to a medae-waewin ceremony. At the time I said, "I'll try anything," but because I was brought up in a strict Catholic faith, I did not want to because of all the things I've heard about the Indian way — it was bad medicine, it was witchcraft, bear-walking and all this.

I really didn't want to go with my sister. But I seen the way she was, how beautiful she walked, the way she looked after her family, the way she walked with her husband and I really admired her. She had been sober for two years and I really admired her. I wanted to be like that. I wanted that life. But it was so hard for me to leave that alcohol alone. I asked her how she did it, and she said by going to hear the old Indian teachings. I said, "I'll try it, I'll do anything."

I had no intention to quit drinking but I went and all the time I was thinking, "Well, they can go to ceremonies and they can drop me off to the nearest bar and they can pick me up on their way back home." They were going there for four days and I t'ought, "Oh, that'd be nice big drunk for me."

But I sure got a surprise when we got there because there was no road to get out. It was about fifteen miles in the bush and I had to stay right there.

There was a healing sweat the second night we were there. I was just terrified because they asked me to go into a sweat and I didn't want to. The person that was conducting that sweat made me sit in the north where that healing comes in. I was just terrified and I wanted to crawl back out of there as soon as that sweat was beginning because it was really dark in there and I didn't know what I was getting myself into.

When I was sittin' in there, it was like, it wasn't a sweat lodge anymore. It was so huge. And I could see this eagle flying around. And this eagle came to me and touched my forehead and stayed with me, sat on my head for a while and just stayed there beside me. I wondered how this eagle got in there. Because everyt'ing is shut and I t'ought that man conducting the sweat must have some kind of powers to do this. It really bothered me but at the same time, I felt good. I felt really good.

I didn't think we were there very long, but we were in there for about three hours. When I came out of there I felt like I wasn't even touching the ground. I felt so light and I felt so good. When I got back to camp I had a hard time falling asleep because I just felt something.

The next day I just wanted to be alone, so I walked towards an opening in the field. Everyone else was getting busy for another ceremony but I just wanted to be alone. I felt like I wanted to cry. I went out in the field near the bush there and I laid down on the ground. I seen four eagles above me. High up in the sky. And I could hear these eagles, "Let go. Let go." I sat up and I looked up and I could hear them. And the four eagles kept circling around until I couldn't see them no more. They just went straight up. And something happened to me. Everything that I did in my life, who I hurt, came flashing in front of me. Especially my daughter and the little boy that I raised. They're the ones I hurt the most.

For the first time in my life, I cried. I cried from within. I never did before. I always cried with self-pity, but I really felt good. And I had a hard, hard time leaving that ceremony because what I found was my identity, who I am as a human being, as a Anishinaubaequae. For the first time I was proud of who I was. For the first time I felt that spirit. I felt really good.

I've never felt like this if I went to church. Even as a child I used to pray so hard and nothing would happen and I would have a hard time trying to believe there was a God. But out here, when I was sitting there and heard those eagles say, "Let go. Let go of everything," I knew the Creator had forgiven me.

When I left there, I never touched a drink for a whole month. But I always, every day, poured myself a drink and poured it back in the bottle. I did this all day long and put the wine back in the fridge.

But I felt really, really lonely, so I left and I went to Sudbury. I went to the bar, to see my friends. I wanted to drink. I asked for a scotch and water but it wouldn't go down. I had to go to the washroom and spit it out because I couldn't even swallow it. It felt like somebody grabbed me by the throat and was choking me. A month later I tried to drink a glass of champagne at my niece's wedding and the same thing happened. The next day I took the bus back to the reserve. I went to see an elder at home and I went crying to him. So he asked me, "What happened to you over there at the ceremony?"

I told him what happened in that sweat lodge. So that old man, he told me, "The Creator helped you. He healed you of your alcoholism. It was Him that was trying to choke you, when you were trying to drink. It was Him that grabbed you by the throat so you wouldn't drink. You were healed. And when that eagle brushed its wings on your forehead, it was telling you that you were getting brain damage from the alcohol and the drugs."

It's true. When I used to be talking, all of a sudden, I'd forget what I was talking about. My mind would just go blank. And I know my hands, if I hold onto a glass or a cup, all of a sudden I'd have no feelings in my fingers. I was always dropping things.

Today I am sober. My life is different. I have a good out-look on life. My family and I are really together today; very, very close. If I was still drinkin' I would never have had this family, my daughter and my three grandchildren. It's the most beautiful gift that has been given to me by the Creator.

I know I got something when I went to that ceremony.

DILA'S STORY

Dila is a fair-skinned forty-nine-year-old Peigan from southern Alberta. She is big, tall and quick to laugh, with a boisterous sense of humour. She is an addictions counsellor and has been sober for eleven years.

When I grew up there was no alcoholism in our fami-ly. My dad used to log and he raised quite a few cattle. We had a pretty decent living. And then in 1964 the liquor opened on the Peigan reserve. I'll never forget the day — April 1, 1964. My dad started to drink and he became chronic. He drank up all his cattle, quit log-ging, just down to nothing. My mother never drank. She ended up going to work. Most of us were grown and married and on our own by then, but they still had five at home.

I didn't fall into drinking right away but everybody else seemed like they just went into it headlong. People were selling their stuff, selling their cows, their horses and it got down to where they were selling their furniture and their appliances. And pretty soon they were selling their shoes and their jackets.

My second husband used to sell everything except his pants. He always liked to wear Levi's and he never sold his pants, but he sold everything else. He'll sell his snap-button shirts, he'll sell his belt and his buckle. He'll sell his boots and he'll sell his jacket and his hat and his wallet and his watch or whatever he had. He'll have nothing and then he'll phone me and he'll say, "I'm real lonesome. I really love you. Can you come and get me?"

And me! I'll just jump in my car and I'll run and get him and I'll bring him home. A couple of times, he was completely sore from head to toe. He had open wounds, what they call wine sores. It took him about a month to heal and I'd be his nurse. I'd be cleaning him, helping him, this and that. And then when he was healthy again, he goes to the employment office, gets a job working in the orchard or something and first payday, he's gone again.

I lived with him for ten years and I'd have to bail him out of jail, go get him in Seattle or Portland or Vancouver. He finally died from cirrhosis in Seattle.

I never went to the bar at first but my first husband used to go. He was always going. Then he started running away with his paycheque and if I chased him and asked him where it is, he'd punch me in the face and beat me up and tell me to get the hell away, he was going to get a new wife, somebody that wasn't so *naggy*.

I didn't like the bars. I used to be scared of them. I used to think that drunks were worse than mentally ill people. I used to think that they didn't know what they were doing. I was real scared of them. My husband would beat me up and the next day he'll say, "I *didn't* even know what I was doing. I didn't even know *a thing*. I didn't even know I beat you up."

That's why I thought that they didn't know what they were doing. But after I started to drink, I find out it's b.s. We know what we're doing. I found out after I tried it myself and I thought, "*You liar*," and I left him. (*laughs*)

After I left him, I got to be really alcoholic. I just lived to go into those bars. I must have been twenty-nine or thirty. I was living with a Mexican and we were living in Yakima, Washington. It was really easy living over there. For an alcoholic it was really a good life, (*laughs*) alcoholic's paradise. You always had these fast jobs you can get. You go work in the orchards, get a few bucks, get drunk, get fired and the next day you go get another job.

When I lived in Seattle we used to live on skid row. We were all winos. I used to get really drunk and go to jail and fight with the police. My favourite line was, "Why don't you just go back to Europe where you belong and leave us alone?" (*laughs*)

It was a lifestyle. It was a total different culture. There was all the blacks, the Chicanos, the Eskimos, the coast Indians and the Plains Indians — Sioux, Cheyenne, Crow, Blackfoot. We were all friends, all the Plains Indians. We all lived together. We were just like a family. We were real close. Somebody would come and say, "So-and-so got beat up last night," and we'd all go over there and visit him and take care of him. We didn't give up and we didn't leave them. We were real true to each other. It was just true brotherhood.

I never worked while I was on skid row but I never got hungry because the guys would go and steal for us. They'd steal whatever we needed. I'd say, "Jeez, I need a change of clothes," and they'd come along with a change of clothes. One time I needed shoes because my heel broke. There were nails sticking out and I was walking on nails and I had blisters all over my heel. I couldn't walk. They went and stole me a pair of shoes.

We always watched each other and at night we'd all huddle together somewhere. It was survival. Like today, if I got a group of men here and we all went and huddled under a tree, they'll probably all want to rape me or something, but not over there. Over there they didn't do those kind of things. And we were protective of them too. We'd really be having a hard time and they'll say, "Why don't you women go rip some guy off?"

And we'd get all fixed up, comb our hair and go uptown to a fancy cocktail lounge and we'll rip off some guy and then go back and give it to them. Whatever we had we always shared.

On skid row we had no money for rent. We didn't have anything. And in 1969, that's the winter I spent on skid row in Seattle, that winter the State cut off all single people over eighteen. I had sent my kids home, so I was classed as single and I didn't get no help. We all managed to get by. We survived.

One year I came home, I think it was 1972, and went to the cemetery and there was sixty new graves. The priest was there and he told me these people all died from alcoholism except two. If there was no alcohol on this reserve, those fifty-eight people would all be still alive. Just a baby and an old man died natural deaths on this reserve that year.

Alcoholism has taken so many lives. Two of my husbands, the two that I was legally married to, are both in the graveyard. The first one drowned in the bathtub; he was having alcohol seizures. And then my second husband, he died in Seattle in 1982 with cirrhosis. My Mexican, he died, got shot. And then I had a boyfriend in Minneapolis and he died too from alcoholism. Jeez, all my husbands are dead and I'm still alive. (*laughs*)

I stayed away for fourteen years and I came back when I heard my first husband died on the reserve back here. So I came back and I couldn't stand the reserve. It was horrible. They didn't have electricity. No plumbing. The wind blew right through the walls. The men were all in jail. They'd go to court for *little* things and they'd give a fifty-dollar fine. At that time fifty dollars was like three or four hundred now and we had no income. People had no jobs. They'd put them in jail. Everybody was just horribly living in poverty. Just *extreme* poverty. I don't know how we ever survived, because there was some kids that died from malnutrition at the time. It was just doom, despair. So I said, "Oh, I gotta get out of here. I can't stand this place."

I moved to Portland, Oregon, and I got a job at the detox centre. I didn't care where I got a job, I just wanted a job. My title was human resources. Gee, I liked my title. It sounded real important. (*laughs*) All I do is go get the food from the catering service and once in a while drive downtown and pick up clients for the centre.

This white woman, my boss, she told me, "Say, do you know the only thing that works for the native people is something called the sweat lodge? We send the blacks, the Chicanos and the whites to a regular treatment centre. But the Indians go into this thing called the sweat lodge and after that we don't see them again, so it must be working. Do you know anything about that?"

I didn't want to be too dumb, so I said, "Yeah, I know about it." I didn't know anything about it. (*laughs*)

I worked there for a while and I came back home. I was the welfare director so I had to watch my behaviour in public. I kind of slowed down on drinking but I still drank. I'd go away to Calgary and I'd get drunk, but I was afraid to drink on the reserve because of my position.

In 1979 we had five suicides in our family. My oldest brother was the first in 1970. And then his oldest son, when he turned nineteen, he shot himself in my dad's house. I wasn't in Brockett too long and my second nephew hung himself. He was nineteen. My mum and dad found him hanging in the barn.

The Catholic priest said in his sermon that God does not forgive suicide. I looked at him and I looked at my nephew in the coffin and I thought, "It just can't be true. I'll believe it for anybody else but not for him. God's gotta forgive him."

So at the graveside I told my younger brother what the priest said. My brother and my fourteen-year-old son had just come from up north. They had went to a place called Faust, Alberta, to this cultural rehabilitation camp.

And my brother said, "We better go back up there, 'cause those people are spiritualists and they communicate with spirits and they'll tell us. The priest doesn't communicate with nobody except his Bible. How do we know that that's true?"

So I said, "Yeah, I guess we better go."

So we got right into that little Datsun and we went up. There was four of us and that's where I met the lady. My son said, "You gotta give her a gift and she'll do a ceremony for you or a sweat lodge tomorrow."

"I don't know what to give her. I got nothing to give her."

And my son said, "You got lots of money. Give her some."

So I looked in my wallet. I found a five. I pulled it out and my son said, "You're too stingy. Give her more."

And I started thinking, "Maybe ten." So I started looking for a ten.

He said, "Give her one of those twenties." And I took real long to pull that twenty out (*laughs*) and I gave it to her.

"Okay," she said, "We'll have a ceremony right now."

I thought, "*Right now*? I'm not even ready." 'Cause in school I was taught you have to clean up before you go to church and here I'm not even clean. It was over a five-hundred-mile drive. So anyway, we had this little ceremony and the spirit did come in and I was scared as could be. I just sat there and shivered through the whole thing and cried. I was sweating and I was trembling and I just didn't know what to do. I was just scared stiff. There was a little kid in there, I just grabbed that kid and I stayed hanging onto that little kid. He didn't even know me; he just let me hang onto him. (*laughs*) That was the first experience I had in native spirituality.

And then the next day we had a sweat lodge. And the same thing. It was really an impact on me. I crawled out of that sweat lodge and I looked around and said, "There is a God and I have found Him."

These evangelists I used to hear on TV saying "rebirth" and "born again," I used to laugh about it and I never thought that it would ever happen to me. And I thought, "This is what's happened to me. I've been reborn. I'm born again."

I was a Christian all my life and I *never* experienced *nothing* like this, not even on Confirmation when they told me the Holy Ghost was gonna blow on me and I was waiting for the Holy Ghost to blow on me and I never felt His breath.

After the sweat lodge was over I asked her, "How does it happen?"

And she said, "Well, it comes through this pipe. It's all through the pipe."

And I said, "Well, if it comes through the pipe and tobacco, then how does it come to the white man?

And she said, "Well, it comes through the wine in the church."

And I said, "You mean to say that the spirit can come through those?"

And she said, "Yes. Different people throughout the world have been given different ways, like the people in the south have been given mescaline and marijuana and peyote, and further south, cocaine. The yellow people use opium in their ceremonies. And the black people have theirs. Every man that's indigenous to land has had a way that God gave him to contact him, and the white man has his wine. And when you use these things outside of the ceremonies, outside of the sacred manner, they become destructive. They destroy people. They're so powerful, once you get addicted to them you have a heck of a time to break away."

And she said, "We have tobacco. Us people have been given tobacco. And tobacco is a killer too. If people use it in a manner of luxury, just to satisfy their physical needs, it's a big killer."

And I said, "Well, what about us drinking around on the street and getting drunk and all that?"

And she said, "Well, the other side comes then."

And, you know, that whole lesson really scared the devil right out of me, and in that one day my life changed. That was the last time I ever drank. I was thirty-eight years old when I finally decided I was reborn.

I never went through treatment, and the basic thing that helped me was the pipe and sweat lodge, eh? But I had to go to psychiatrists too. A lot of my problems stem from low self-esteem and lack of self-worth. I had a horrible inferiority complex with white people. I just hated all white people because I thought I couldn't be one of them or I couldn't be like them or I thought they were better than me. And people used to tell me, "Why do you hate white people when you just look like one of them?" That was a real big insult.

I believe that alcoholism among native people is a cover-up for all the wrongs where we've been dehumanized by the white society. You just name it and they took it. They took our rights. They took our land. They took the resources. They're polluting the land, the rivers, the air.

They took away our brains 'cause they brainwashed us in the boarding schools. They took away our language. They took away our songs. They outlawed our ceremonies. They outlawed parts of the sundance back, I think, in 1916. The last man that pierced in the sundance ceremony went to jail and then everybody was scared after that and there was no more piercing. They couldn't fast to do their vision quest. It was against the law too. They just whipped our spirits. It's the emotional part and the spiritual part that they hit on so hard.

In 1982 I think it was, I went back to Seattle and started to look for my friends. I found one and asked him, "Where's so-and-so and so-and-so and so-and-so?"

"Oh, he was pretending to rob a hotel and the clerk thought he had a gun 'cause he had his hand in his jacket like this and he shot him. And then so-and-so was found in an alley. He was dead. Another guy, somebody threw him down a stairwell in a hotel right down to the bottom. Another one got thrown out of a fifth-storey window. Another one was climbing into his own apartment on the fourth floor, he was drunk, and the police saw him and they hollered to stop and he didn't and they shot him."

They were just all dead.

Around here they have this program called the Adult Children of Alcoholics. The first time I went in the program I thought, "That's not for me 'cause my parents didn't drink when I was growing up."

But when I looked at the symptoms of it, I thought, "Geez, that's me. I think I got like that in boarding school 'cause the rules of Adult Children of Alcoholics was 'Don't trust, don't feel.' "

And those are exactly what I was brought up with. When I first went to school, I'd cry and they'd slap me around and say, "Quit crying, you crybaby." So pretty soon I learned that I shouldn't have those kind of feelings. Or if you're too happy, "You're being too silly. You're being too ridiculous." We'd get punished if we were too happy or too sad, so we had to be always just on the line.

And how could we trust them when we knew we couldn't tell them our real truth? I remember there was a sundance going on and a nun said, "Don't partake in that sundance over there 'cause the devil is over there and it's black magic and it's voodoo. And if you go over there, the priest is going to excommunicate you."

My grandfather was over there but I couldn't say anything. I just had to look at her and I thought, "Those people at the sundance are a lot better than you. They're kinder than you. They're more generous than you. Everything is better about them."

How can a little kid trust somebody like that?

It was really (*sighs*) dehumanizing in so, so many ways. They're always so ready to punish. We all had to dress the same. We all had to cut our hair the same. We all had to eat the same time. We were *forever* praying and mumbling a bunch of Latin. I never knew what I was saying and we'd spend hours saying it, plus singing it.

I think those are the things that caused alcoholism to have such a toll on the people today. I think once the Indian people have their identity back, it's gonna be a better time for us. But the problem is how to get it back because some of them are so badly brainwashed it's *really* difficult. All they see is the material side of life and a lot of them will sell out because there's so much poverty.

To understand our native culture, we have to understand spirituality, because native culture is based on spirituality. And we can't understand spirituality if we're brainwashed, so we have to become (*laughs*) debrainwashed. That's not an easy thing.

In 1979, that was the first time in my life I went into a sweat lodge. I didn't have any kind of understanding of my own culture. I didn't know a Indian song or the meaning of the songs. I just thought it was a lot of noise and a lot of banging. I didn't understand it at all.

But yet the feeling was there, like when I smelled that sweetgrass, I thought of my grandfather. It took me back to my early childhood where my grandfather used to set up a tipi and he had a ceremony that he did with a pipe to welcome the thunder in the spring and then in the falltime the same ceremony to send the thunder back. I didn't understand it at all, but we used to participate in it. He'd be sitting up by the fire there and he'd call us over one by one and he'd paint our faces with red ochre. And then in the mornings they used to get up real early and go out and pray when the morning star appeared and the rising of the sun.

I think what really helped me was native spirituality 'cause from that day to now I haven't drunk. That's eleven years ago. And my children all don't drink now 'cause each one of them came into the sweat lodge.

Now we have a sweat lodge back home, up in the hills, and there's a group of people that's going there and they're not drinking. A lot of the people that I know have went back to their own spirituality and there's sobriety with them. It's really helped my family. And I've seen a lot of other Indian people that have been helped by it. Probably if I didn't go up north and go to that sweat lodge, I'd be dead by now.

10

Treatment

"The people in the treatment cracked the iceberg that I was and I began to melt after being three days in the hotseat."

Native people who want to deal with their alcoholism through a residential treatment program have a number of options. They can, like anyone else, enter a public treatment centre. Most native people, however, go to one of the fifty treatment centres across Canada that are operated by and for native people. Most of these centres are financed by Health and Welfare Canada and provide a treatment program based, in large part, on the twelve-step self-help philosophy of Alcoholics Anonymous. The treatment programs usually have a large measure of local native culture, as well. In a few places, the treatment program is conducted in the local native language.

Most of the staff at native treatment centres are native people who are recovering alcoholics. They have to deal with the same stress as that faced by public treatment centre workers, but they must also face the additional stress that comes from playing a visible and sometimes unpopular role in a small community. So despite their good work and good intentions, addictions workers and native treatment centres are sometimes subject to harsh criticism from community members.

RON is a moody, dark-skinned forty-four-year-old Metis. An oil industry engineer, Ron has been sober since he left a public treatment centre in Saskatchewan two and a half years ago.

I was a social drinker. I'd get plastered once in a while on ski trips and fishing trips. Seemed normal, working in a high-stress profession. Everyone needs to let their hair down once in a while and get away from it all. Don't they?

At my very worst I drank about two dozen beer a week. I had more of an ego problem than a drinking problem. Drugs were more of a problem with me.

I had to see a psychologist because I was coming unglued, mentally and emotionally. They sent me to detox and to a treatment centre at Estevan.

When I was in detox I read this paper called the disease concept of alcoholism, and I became convinced that I was alcoholic. The definition was "a chronic progressive incurable disease characterized by loss of control over alcohol and other drugs."

By that definition I said, "Yeah. I sure as hell have lost control of something."

I'd really lost control of my thinking, which is pretty easy to do when you got a whole bunch of psycho-active drugs working on your brain. I don't care who you are. Give him a little bit of booze every day and give him sleeping pills at night and Valium every morning and that guy's gonna have a problem.

When I ended up in detox I found myself sitting there in this group of people and everybody was sitting there saying, "My name is so-and-so and I'm an alcoholic."

I was in such a mental state that if everybody had been sitting there saying, "My name is so-and-so and I'm a pumpkin pie," I would have said, "My name's Ron and I must be a pumpkin pie too."

That's the kind of distress I was in at that time and that's when I first said, "Yeah, I'm an alcoholic."

Estevan was a very good program except that I got asked to leave on the twenty-third of twenty-eight days. They told me I was not ready for treatment. They told me that I was not alcoholic. They told me that all I had was an ego, a control and a trust problem.

I was hurt. I was very confused and hurt. I did not want to go because the following Tuesday I was scheduled to take my fifth step in this twelve-step program. The fifth step says that we have to admit to God, to ourselves and to another human being the exact nature of our wrongs. And I know now just how vital that fifth step is to come to terms with me and the way I related to the people around me. I did not want to go. I just about got down on my knees and begged my counsellor to let me stay to do that fifth step.

So I thought like, "What is wrong with me? If I'm not an alcoholic, what the hell is my problem?"

I was very confused. I felt really lost. I wasn't angry. I was much relieved if anything knowing that I did not have that illness. I had no idea what to do next. None. They just said, "There's a bus leaving at seven o'clock tonight. Be on it. We'll let you back in ninety days."

They must have thought I had some more drinking to do to become alcoholic and *then* they'd let me back. That's the only reason I can figure. (*sighs*) I knew I had a problem and I knew it was not fully treated by any stretch of the imagination.

D.L.S. is a thirty-seven-year-old Chippewa woman who grew up in southern Ontario. She sobered up in a public treatment centre in British Columbia two years ago.

In April of 1988, I entered treatment for the third time — the Maple Ridge treatment centre — and it was in there that something cracked the iceberg that was me. I've never experienced before what I experienced there.

It was run by white people, by recovered alcoholics, and I was the only native person there. When I got there, I made a quick assessment that I knew better than most of the clients, because I had had some experience in treatment as well as some exposure to AA, and I felt the staff couldn't tell me anything that I didn't know.

But I had to go on this hotseat for three days and the little group that I was put in had a few hard drug addicts, one housewife, a couple of ironworkers, myself and this police officer who had a specialty in interrogation. And when I was on the hotseat they wanted us to tell the story of our life, starting from where we were born. So I began to tell them the story of my life and I guess I was moving rather rapidly and they would stop me and want to know details. They told me that I told my history like I was reading from a textbook and they accused me of displaying no emotion whatsoever.

Of course I got very defensive and very angry, and I said, "You had to be there to appreciate what went on." And it was during the hotseat time that I came in touch with the anger and, more importantly, with the pain of my life.

I am the third-eldest of fourteen children. I come from a very rigid religious background. My father got religion when I was five years old but we experienced a lot of abuse, a lot of physical, a lot of emotional, a lot of mental and sexual abuse. I always walked around carrying secrets because I didn't want people to know what really happened to me. I never really got in touch with all the pain that I had lived through as a child, as a teenager.

So the people in the treatment cracked the iceberg that I was and I began to melt after being three days on the hot-seat. For the first time, I saw the effects of my alcoholism on my child, who is now eighteen years of age. I just was flooded with tears, that I could have done all that I done to that poor little girl. That's when I began to open up.

In my mind, I went in there, well, intact, and I came out of there sick. Now I'm beginning to try to recover in the recovery program. I have been clean for two years, but it's been very painful.

SANNGIJUQ is a twenty-nine-year-old inuk with delicate features and long black hair. She has been sober for nine months. She was interviewed on a park bench in Ottawa.

I went to a treatment centre called Bellwood Health Services in Toronto to quit drinking. I detested the treatment program. I thought the staff was obnoxious and fakes. I thought there was a catch to all this being friendly, that's what I thought of the program. I thought that they were snobbish and real fakes in being kind.

It was run by different people. There was one Chinese counsellor and one from Egypt, Iran or whatever. There were a lot of white people.

I had a lot of problems 'cause I was really the only native who was there out of about forty to fifty people — staff and clients together. I was the only inuk. I thought I was too different because my skin is dark, my hair is black. I thought, "Well, I'll change if I dye my hair blonde. Why can't I be with the 'in' group?" I even discussed it with my group therapy and I realized, like, "I'm fine," you know? I don't have to be with the "in" group anymore.

I had a lot of problems. The hardest thing was to actually open up and talk about how I'm feeling. Whenever a counsellor or therapist or a client asked me, "So how are you feeling?" I would go, "Oh, I'm just the quiet type, that's all." But here I was hurting and angry, sad and guilty.

I changed my opinion of the staff because of the patience they had — the genuine and sincere caring, kindness and understanding for me. You know, a couple of them cried with me, hugged me. They were very, very patient and understanding and opened up my eyes and ears to looking at life in such a different way. I didn't want to leave them. The day I graduated I was hoping one of the staff would come up and say to me, "You cannot leave us." But of course they didn't 'cause they knew I had to let go of them.

They were the most sincerest and genuine, kind understanding people I ever met. They were absolutely beautiful people.

ALLAN is a no-nonsense twenty-five-year-old Peigan. He has been sober for three years and is an addictions counsellor on the Blood reserve in southern Alberta. His office walls are covered with inspirational posters.

The toughest part of my job is when an individual has been through the grind, has hit rock bottom and knows that they might die because of alcoholism and says "no" to help.

I had a client one time knew he was gonna die because of alcoholism but kept drinking and drinking and I just waited, just sat here wondering, "Where is he? When will he finally kick the bucket?" I think sometimes that is the hardest part of the job for me.

You see a lot of people come in with the shakes, dehydrated, their lives going down the drain. I just finished talking to an individual who has hit rock bottom. This guy has been kicked around, his clothes look like they've been on for about a week. He hasn't taken a good shower for maybe longer than that, and you've got to show this individual that there's a good life other than alcoholism? When their mother and father have just passed away? They got no job, nothing to look forward to. Their family doesn't want them. And you gotta show this person that there's a better way of living than what they're living right now?

He's thirty-five years old and he can't understand how I quit drinking. I told him, "It comes from here (*pounds his chest*) and a lot of praying."

But those people look at me and say, like, "Who the hell do you think you are sobering up and showing off and everything like that?"

Sometimes I've had a few individuals that came up to me and have did that, but in our training, you tend to put something in front of you, a mirror-type thing. So they're not really yelling at you, they're yelling at themselves, saying, "Why can't I do that?"

They come up and they call me names. They shoot a lot of garbage at me. They call down my family, especially me, but then I put this mirror-thing in front of me and it's not me they're calling down. They're fighting within themselves.

KATE is a sixty-three-year-old Blackfoot elder from southern Alberta. She is a large woman with curly white hair. She speaks slowly, with a measured calmness. She has been sober for twenty-six years and is an addictions counsellor at a native treatment centre.

I've helped a lot of people to quit drinking since I came to sober up myself. I know how much I suffered, so I know how much the people suffer and it helps me to get concerned and to have feelings for them, to want them to find what I have found.

I lost many cases, many people I couldn't get to because they didn't want to respond. There's a lot that I have helped that were ready. They were tired of drinking and living that way and they wanted to change and I just kind of give them a helping hand and they sobered up.

There was one woman I helped; she had cirrhosis like me. She was sober for a year and then she fell off and she went back to drinking. She drank for just three weeks and she died. That really disappointed me. I didn't want to help nobody anymore 'cause I was so hurt. I felt that I should have been with her more often, 'cause I was sponsoring her and I kind of felt guilty that I wasn't there when she fell off.

I didn't want to help anybody anymore after that, but people came to me and I started over again. Today I don't get frustrated anymore if people don't quit drinking 'cause I understand that I can't run other people's lives. I can only run mine. I help where I can and if they want it, it's there. And if they don't, it's their choice.

You stick with the ones that are trying. But the main one is me. I've got to look after me. That's what I've learned.

MARK is a forty-six-year-old Mohawk. Tall, rugged and strong-featured with braided hair hanging halfway down his back, he spits out his words in a tough, deadpan delivery. He quit drinking, with no outside help, twenty years ago. He was interviewed on the banks of the Grand River in southern Ontario.

It's a *disgrace* to have alcohol and drug abuse centres in Indian territories. These are all white organizations. People have become so white-minded they figure it's the only way to go. The reason I say a treatment centre shouldn't be here is because as native people we should help each other. We should be willing to help a person that needs counselling, in your home, or like we're setting here now, by the river. We should be able to meet as people, as human beings, not as some organization. Everybody has to get involved. It can't be just a *committee* set up. That's *white* mentality. That's *white* thinking.

These alcohol and drug abuse centres, everything that they do revolves around money. It don't revolve around compassion. They don't want to see alcohol and drug abuse end because the people that run those things are out of a job then. They're gettin' paid and that's wrong. I don't think there should be any payment have to be made for helpin' a brother or a sister get away from alcohol or drugs. I think the payment is just seein' that they don't do it anymore. That's payment enough.

For twenty years I've been sober and different people have asked me what they can do, how can they stop. And all you can do is sit down and relate your story to them because it's gotta come from inside themselves to get away from that.

I always tell them it's not our heritage to drink. We got to get back to the basic way of Indian thinking. We incorporate too much of the white way of thinking and that don't cure things. It just *prolongs* things.

❦

ROY'S STORY

Roy is a thirty-eight-year-old Dene from the Northwest Territories. He is a huge man with a large stomach. He wears his waist-length black hair in a pony tail and has a wispy moustache and a soft, breathy voice. He was interviewed in a native treatment centre where he was training to become an addictions counsellor.

The whole idea of drinking was easy to get into because my father was an alcoholic and I grew up in a community where everybody was drinking except for three or four women. Everybody else in that community used to drink a lot.

A while ago I was watching a TV program and this girl didn't want to bring any of her friends home because her mother was an alcoholic. So she'd make up some lame excuse that something was happening at her house so they could never do homework there 'cause she was too ashamed of her mother.

I remember looking at that and thinking it was never that way for us. I seen my father passed out quite a bit and I remember people bringing him home or I'd pick him up off the street and bring him home. I was never ashamed of him.

Like if somebody passed out anywhere, all the kids would get together and we'd pick them up and go knocking on somebody's door and say, "Hey, your father's drunk," or "Your husband's drunk," and bring them in and throw them on the bed. We enjoyed bringing people home. That was a good time to hit our parents up for money, like when they were feeling generous and carefree. Ask them for a buck and they'd give it to you. So you'd make sure you brought your friends home then.

And if a couple of guys were drinking and fighting, to us, it was a show. It was fun to see these guys and then the next day to watch these guys try to make up for what they did to each other the day before. These kind of things would happen all the time. Like, to us, it was just normal.

But my mother never touched a drop in her life. I thought my mother was weird. I grew up thinking there was something wrong with my mum 'cause she never drank.

I remember when I was younger one of my aunts asked my brother if he was ever gonna drink and he said "no." And I remember she asked me and I proudly looked at her and I said "yes." And I did. (*laughs*) I drank for almost ten years, I guess. I drank quite heavily.

The thing that I really enjoyed about drinking was that it gave me a lot of confidence that I never had before. I had a real low self-esteem, and drinking just made me feel good about myself and I was able to say and do things that I couldn't do when I was sober.

I really enjoyed drinking. I had a good time when I drank. But when I blacked out I got into fights and there was times when I got beat up quite badly. And there was times when I'd wake up and I'd find blood on my shirt and I don't remember whose blood it is, whether it's my own or somebody else's. These were the scary parts.

I liked drinking so much I just did it all the time. I don't know how I survived school, like I dropped out of school when I was in grade nine and I decided to go back when I was nineteen and take upgrading. I went to a place in Fort Smith, to an adult education centre there and, oh, there used to be a lot of drinking going on. Like to this day I don't know how I survived those three years, because I drank quite a bit. There was quite a few times I woke up in the drunk tank or passed out on somebody's floor or passed out in a ditch somewhere. And yet I did really well in school, and today I think, "Boy, I did well while I was drinking. I wonder how good I would have done if I had stayed sober, eh?"

I finished my schooling and I got a job, but then I was drinking heavily. I was right into it. Like there was money in my pocket all the time and that's all I did. I drank my money. Sometimes I wouldn't eat for two or three days 'cause I had drunk up all my money. But I didn't mind that. I just felt that was the thing to do.

I moved into this one community and all I did was drink. I lived there for almost a year when I met a lady, a woman that eventually I married and I'm still with her today. It's funny how we met, like one day I was partying at this guy's house and we were really whooping it up. I blacked out and when I came to, I was sleeping at the end of a couch in somebody else's house at the other end of town and there was somebody else sleeping at the other end of the couch. I found a case of beer on the floor and I opened a bottle because I was feeling so terrible I had to drink in order to feel better. While I was moving around, this lady woke up and she introduced herself to me and I introduced myself to her and I married her a year later.

On my wedding day there was a reception and everybody started drinking a lot and I got in a fight with someone and I ended up in jail on my wedding night. (*laughs*) The next day I woke up in the drunk tank and they let me out and I went home and I started drinking again. And again I got drunk that night and I passed out, so I didn't sleep with my wife till the third night. (*laughs*) That's how bad it was for me.

I used to work all the time and I'd go and buy a radio or tape recorder or camera or something and first drunk, I'd go broke and I used to go hock them all the time. I used to sell all my stuff, so I never really owned anything. When I got married, all I had was the shirt on my back, my clothes and a stereo that wasn't fully paid for. That's all I owned when I got married.

After I got married my wife became pregnant and she didn't want to drink when she was pregnant, so she quit. But I kept partying.

This one time, I got drunk and she was so mad at me that she pushed me and I fell down and I was so drunk I couldn't even get off the floor. I just passed out and she left me there. And the next morning I was angry. I had a vague memory of her pushing me and me falling down and I couldn't get up and I was really angry. I was so mad at her, I slapped her and she threw me out of the house. I was still drunk when I did that. Then I thought, "The hell with you," and I took off to my home community, which was about a hundred miles away.

When I was growing up I remember my father beating up my mother and I never thought I would touch a woman. I did, and boy, I was ashamed of that. I didn't go home for a week or so and finally I got enough guts and I phoned her. She told me, "You can come home whenever you want. I know you were drunk. Come home whenever you're ready." So I did eventually. I went back.

I didn't drink for a while because of what I had did to my wife, so I promised myself I wasn't gonna drink while my wife was pregnant. A few months later a little baby was born, but again there was another reason for celebration. I saved up some money and I planned this party after my son was born for the long weekend in August. I went to my home community 'cause there was no liquor store where we were living and I brought back this whole load of booze. And of course I got carried away and I don't remember hardly anything for the next three or four days.

I remember waking up on a Tuesday morning. We were living in this little house, not very big. In fact, it was my mother-in-law's 'cause I didn't own nothing. My mother-in-law was good enough to let us live with her. We had a little two-bedroom shack. She lived in one bedroom and we lived in the other one.

I remember I was laying there and I was waking up, you know, and this noise was coming at me and it was really bothering me 'cause I was just sicker than a dog. I was just so sick. This noise was bothering me and I didn't want to wake up. But eventually I sat up in bed and kind of shake the cobwebs out of my mind, trying to figure out where was that noise coming from. And all of a sudden I realized it was a baby crying. I wanted him to quit crying because he was giving me a headache.

You know, (*sighs*) to this day, I think you could have took a two-by-four and hit me on the head and tell me to quit drinking, it wouldn't have helped. But that moment. I got up and I walked up to the crib and I think I sobered up that moment when I saw the baby kicking around in his mess. I didn't know when the last time was we cleaned him. And he was just screaming, he was so miserable.

I always promised myself as a young man that I would never get married. I would never have any kids. But I did get married and I had this kid. And that morning when I woke up and I stood there by the bed, my whole life flashed before my eyes. And how hopeless I felt at times and how I used to watch people drinking and getting hurt and I used to watch people beating each other up and all these things all of a sudden came rushing back in at that one moment. And I thought, "God, I can't do this to my son. I can't do this to my little baby." I wanted my baby to have a good life, I wanted him to grow up feeling good about himself. I wanted him to grow up to be proud that he is a human being.

And at that moment, it hit me so damn hard. I had some booze left over and I went and dug up all that booze. My wife was still sleeping and I took all that booze, and we didn't even have an inside toilet, we just had an outhouse, and I went out there and I dumped all the booze. And I never drank again. I didn't want to touch any alcohol. I wanted to give my child a good life. So I quit drinking.

You know, (sighs) I think that was the best thing I ever did for myself but, unfortunately I didn't know about the AA program. I quit drinking in 1977 when my son was born. And I went to a treatment program in April 1989. So that was twelve years that I was sober, not drinking. But all my attitudes and the whole idea of being a dry drunk was with me.

I used to gamble lots. I became an overeater. I worked like a bastard. I started working with my band in 1978 and I remember working until five, six o'clock in the morning, sitting in my office and typing. All of a sudden I'd come to, and I'd look at my watch and it's five o'clock in the morning. I'd go home, have a couple hours' sleep and be back at work at eight or nine o'clock.

And I chased bingos like crazy. I'd drive six hundred miles for a bingo. My wife and I chased bingos all over the countryside. Like I lived in Hay River and I went to Fort Smith for bingo. I went to Pine Point, Fort Resolution, Yellowknife on a few occasions. I even came down to Edmonton for bingo. And bingo wasn't enough. I got into playing poker and I used to play poker like crazy.

And I thought I was happy. I was sober and having a good life. But during those years my self-esteem was really bad. I was really miserable.

I worked for my band as a band manager and I tried to get the band to look at what it was doing, 'cause I really felt that alcohol was hurting our people and I felt, "If I can sober up, they can do it. All they got to do is put their mind into it and sober up and everything will be okay."

I really believed that if I could sober my people up, things would be a lot better. I pushed and pushed and pushed and some people would sober up for a while and then go back to drinking and then I'd feel so defeated. And then if they did sober up they would have some other addiction and would be neglecting their children.

I thought, "Well, if they had good houses they'll be okay." So we started encouraging the band to build good houses. And if they had good jobs, they'll be okay. And I went out and created all kinds of jobs, but the people were still just as miserable as ever. I thought I was doing the right thing. I was going through life thinking that if I can build good houses for my people they'll sober up. If I gave them a good job, they'll want to stay sober. And I chased that for a long time.

But during that time I was really pushing myself. For twelve years I pushed and pushed and pushed and eventually I had a breakdown. I fell apart emotionally. I couldn't cope with things. By March 1989 I was at the end of my rope. I was just going crazy. I didn't understand what was happening to me. I thought there was something wrong with these other people. I thought I was okay.

I had my breakdown just about two weeks after this friend of mine got back from treatment. She pulled me aside and said, "Hey, Roy, there's something wrong with you. What you need is to go for treatment."

At the beginning I was thinking, "What the hell is she talking about?" You know? "She's the one with the problem, I haven't drunk for twelve years. I got no problem."

But she didn't say, "You're an alcoholic." She told me, "Roy, there's something happening to you that you don't understand and you need to deal with it. Why don't you go for treatment?"

"What the hell is she talking about? I'm not an alcoholic. I didn't drink for twelve years. I'm healthy. I got no problem. She's the one with the goddam alcohol problem."

That was my immediate reaction. It took two hours for her to make me realize that I was sick. Eventually she said, "Look, Roy, Poundmaker's is a place of healing. It's a place for you to take care of yourself and if you went there, you would be able to heal yourself."

By then I was really miserable and really desperate. I knew there was something wrong. Like all my fingertips were all raw. My nerves were all shot. I had gained probably over a hundred pounds in a matter of a year. And physically I wasn't doing well.

She told me, "Look, you got to go for treatment. Even just to go on a break."

That's when I said, "Okay." I said, "I'm gonna go to Poundmaker's to take a break. I'm gonna take a holiday."

I came here on March 29, 1989. I didn't want to waste people's time, so I thought I'm really gonna get into this thing and I'm really gonna try for twenty-eight days. I can get away from politics and get away from my family for twenty-eight days and I can just take a good rest.

First thing they did was they hand me a Step One book, you know, to go through the AA program. They handed me a book and I looked at it. "I'm not an alcoholic. What the hell are you doing?"

But I felt guilty about wasting other people's time, so I thought I better put on a good show. At least I should try. So I went through that step and I answered all the questions and I handed in the book and the next day the counsellor brought that back and said, "You got to do this over."

I went, "What the hell you mean, I got to do it over?"

I couldn't understand what he was talking about. I answered all the questions about my life becoming unmanageable. For example, a question might have said, "What shameful things would you have done while you were drinking? Name two or three times when you had blacked out." I answered them, but I guess I didn't answer them right.

So I did it over a second time and I handed it in and again that bugger brought it back to me and he said, "You didn't do this right. You're not being honest with yourself. You're not accepting that you're an alcoholic."

And I thought "Goddam that guy. What's he doing?" You know? "Why is he trying to make me an alcoholic? I'm not." Like I was really convinced I had no alcohol problem.

He handed me back my step booklet again and he said, "Look, we really want you to try and look back. Look back during your drinking years. Don't answer these questions because you want to get through the book. Sit down and think of moments that you can remember and it's gonna be hard for you because it was twelve years ago that you drank. But remember what it did to you and how you felt at those times."

And I did. I really honestly sat down and started working on it. And you know, I admitted I was an alcoholic. 'Cause back then I had no control over it. Alcohol completely controlled my life. I started remembering these things and I was just sick when I admitted that I was an alcoholic. Like I was just really devastated with the idea that I was an alcoholic. Up to then I thought I was in control. And yet I wouldn't touch a drop because I was too scared of it. I couldn't accept the fact that there was something that controlled me.

But the next step eased my pain. I had to accept a higher power to bring me back to sanity. And, boy, that one was a real saver for me. In Step Three, they talk about turning your will and your life over to the higher power, as we understood Him. I couldn't understand that.

What the hell did that mean? You know? Why did God give me my will if I'm going to give it back to Him? That doesn't make sense.

I was struggling with that and one day we were sitting in the ceremonial circle and the elder was speaking and he said, "All these things that you did during your drinking years, all these shameful things in your past — God can take that all away from you. All you have to do is hand it over to Him. And He'll take care of it."

At that time I was just mentally in a mess. I had all these crazy ideas about my people and I thought, "I can help my people. *I* can make them better." I, I, I, I. All they have to do is listen to *me*. If they can listen to me, I can help them. That's the idea I had.

I was sitting there and all of a sudden I understood what they meant by turning your will and your life over to the power of God and to humble yourself. All of a sudden I understood, because up to that moment I tried to control the world. I tried to do it my way. I didn't worry if there was a God. And every time something happened I took responsibility for it. You know. And I remember I was sitting there and I thought, "Oh, my God. Now I understand. I understand."

And I prayed and I said, "God, You have me. You got me where You want me. I'm tired of doing what I do. I'm tired of trying to control everyone. It's not up to me. It's not my responsibility. It's Yours and I'm gonna give it to You. You do what You have to in my life."

And in that moment I turned my will and my life over to the power of God and it was just like the whole world was lifted off my shoulder. I walked out of that ceremonial circle and I walked outside and the first thing I saw was the sunlight. In all my life I never, ever *saw* the sunlight. I didn't know it was there. I took it for granted. I went and I sat outside in the sunlight. I was sitting there and enjoying the sunlight for the first time in my life. I remember I was feeling so good. And this guy walked up to me and he said, "Aren't you Roy?"

I looked at him and I was surprised. Why was he asking me that? And I said, "Yeah, I'm Roy."

He said, "You look so different. What happened to you?"

"What do you mean, what happened to me?"

You know, I think he saw my spirit in a different light. To this day I remember that really well, that feeling of euphoria. You know. And I didn't have to take a high to get it. For once in my life I felt so good about myself. I felt so good that I was alive. I felt so good that I wasn't responsible for anybody else in this world but myself.

Eventually I got through the program and when I went home I realized I couldn't be a chief anymore 'cause I was working against all the principles of the AA program and all the principles of me being sober. But I decided not to resign and I stayed on.

The three or four months after I came out of treatment, I just struggled from day to day because everything I remember doing, like giving houses free to our people, is wrong. You know, we're taking the responsibility away. We bitch and complain as Indian people that our control had been taken away from us and that the government owes us everything. Just handing things free to our people is not right, because all we've turned into is Indian agents. Like that's what I felt like. I just felt like an Indian agent. My band members were coming to me and asking me for things and I was giving it to them. It wasn't right. And it felt so self-defeating. Like it was just going against all the principles of my sobriety.

Someday I hope all our people come to the realization what alcohol is doing to them. It's not the government that's doing it to us anymore. We're doing it to ourselves through alcohol. Like some people are doing economic development and I believe that that's the answer. Somehow we have to turn our lives around and take responsibility for ourselves. I really believe that the government can only do so much for us. Like sure, they're going to hand us money, but let's use it in a positive way. Like here, Poundmaker's is a positive way of taking government money and making it work for our people. Rather than just as a handout. Who in the heck feels good about being handed something for free? You know? I really believe in what we're doing here in Poundmaker's — healing people and bringing up their spirit and getting them to understand themselves as human beings.

But then something happened and I had a relapse. I didn't go back to drinking, but I went back to my old way of thinking. I really thought that I could change things, you know. I could change the government's mind. If I could just go at it full tilt, I can change things.

So that's what I did. I chased land claims. I was with the Dene Nation land claims for six months. I stood in the front line with the negotiators. I became the negotiator and I lost myself in that. I put everything into that. Like my whole energy went into land claims.

And at the end of it we had nothing. I didn't agree with the signing. Like, to me, I felt we did our best and this was the best we can offer our people, so we may as well accept it. But anyway, the land claims was over and June 20th was band elections and I didn't run again for chief.

I'm free now. I don't feel obligated that I have to do something for my people. I feel that I can help them but I don't feel that same kind of a misguided idea about what my people need. I just got to take care of myself and live my life the best I can and if I can set an example for somebody else to begin the process of recovery from alcoholism or drugs, if I can encourage that in one individual, then I've done good.

I feel good about myself today. I'm happy. I'm happy to be alive and I'm happy to be sober. And finally — finally — I'm starting to heal. I'm starting to get over the hurts I went through as a child, all the pain and the shame and the gut feelings from my drinking days. I'm starting to heal. I'm beginning to feel like a human being.

Like I was a chief, a band manager, I was all these things. That's what I *was*. I didn't understand *me*. I lived from right here (*points at his neck*) up. I knew all the problems in the world. Like if you ask me a question about Russia, the United States, anything in this world,

I had an opinion and I had it all figured out. But if you ever ask about *me*, Roy, "Hey, how do you feel right now?" I couldn't tell you. I didn't know.

Today I can tell you. I can tell you what's happening here. (*points to his heart*) Now I can say I'm frustrated, I'm angry, feeling low. I understand those feelings now. Before I couldn't get into that. Like, don't feel. Don't trust. Don't talk. That's something that really had me by the balls and that's the way I lived my life.

Today I realize that I've got a lot of acquaintances, but I don't have any friends. And that's fucking scary, man. That blows me fucking away. You know? Knowing that I've got no friends. Because they didn't know me. There was nothing they knew about me. Every time somebody got too close to me, I ran. I don't know how the heck I got married.

I quit running away 'cause now I know it wasn't those other people that was doing it to me. I was doing it to myself and I used to blame everybody for it. Now I don't blame anybody for my problems. If I got a problem, I created it.

I still struggle every day. I go through a lot of emotions every day. At least I can deal with them now. So when Mulroney starts pissing me off, I start thinking, "Why am I thinking that way? Why am I responding this way to this guy?" Before I just didn't understand that.

I don't know how things are going to be tomorrow. I take it one day at a time. I don't have to prove nothing anymore. I'm not the centre anymore. I'm just a part of this whole universe. So that's my story.

11

ALCOHOLICS ANONYMOUS

"AA is the answer. It's very open. It doesn't refer to any nationality. It applies to anybody. It's not just for white people."

An alcoholic, according to the definition of Alcoholics Anonymous, is someone who is powerless to control his or her craving for alcohol. To AA, alcoholism is a disease, and the only cure is complete abstention, combined with spiritual renewal.

Alcoholics Anonymous has been enormously successful, all by itself, in helping thousands of native people recover from alcoholism. In addition, the twelve-step self-help principles of AA have been adopted by almost all fifty native treatment centres as the basis of their programs. Many native people credit AA's success to the fact that it is open to all races and flexible enough to allow for the expression and inclusion of native cultural practices and spiritual beliefs.

Alcoholics Anonymous is not without critics and limitations, however. For example, many native people do not have the level of education necessary to use or benefit from its literature. As well, AA's formal structures and procedures repel many native people in remote northern communities.

CHRISTINE is a twenty-eight-year-old Nisga'a from the Naas valley in northern British Columbia. Short, smiling and filled with bubbly good cheer, she has been sober for four years. She was interviewed in a Vancouver hotel room.

I've never been to a treatment centre. I quit drinking mostly through the AA program and that's really helped me a lot. The AA program was loving, it was fun. It was great. It was exciting. It was new. The people accepted me. They treated me *equal*. They didn't ask me questions. They didn't care where I came from. They didn't care what I had done, just that I stay sober.

AA is a part of my life. It's an everyday thing. It's something I have to work on on a daily basis and I will never complete this program. It keeps me sober and if I want to stay sober, that's where I have to go. I've been sober for four years and I want to *die* sober. But I have to do it one day at a time. There was a time where I had to think to myself, "I will make it by this restaurant without going in and having a drink." I do it with that restaurant and I do it with the next restaurant I pass. It took everything I had to stay sober. And it worked. It's not just one day at a time. It's one *step* at a time sometimes. I will just keep one foot going in front of the other and get myself to a meeting. One step at a time.

BETTY is a middle-aged Metis. A husky-voiced chain smoker, she sobered up with the help of AA thirteen years ago. She is a counsellor with an inner-city neighbourhood organization in Edmonton.

AA is the answer. It's very open. If you read the book, Chapter Five, that's where it tells you how it works. It's all there, Chapter Five. That's where I found my direction. It talks about *me* and how I can change my life and how I can be responsible for me. It doesn't talk about anything else. It doesn't refer to any nationality. It applies to anybody. It's not just for white people.

AA, to me, is like the culture. I was raised very spiritually, very traditionally and my dad taught me all these things that I've been taught in AA. I've been taught to share, to care. I practised all these things when I was child — to respect, to be honest. I was taught all them things as a child. I lost them all through alcohol, and AA has given me that back.

AA is a very spiritual program, that's what I like about it. The first two steps talk about alcohol, and the rest are all about change — changing oneself and coming to believe in a higher power. I lost that belief. AA has given me that back. Like I believe strongly in the Great Spirit and I got that back through AA. It's not that I never had it, it's that I lost it through my alcoholism.

There was the love and the sharing and the caring that they practise in AA — we had that before. We had it when we lived in the bush. We had that strength, we had that power. We didn't need alcohol back then to enjoy ourself.

A long time ago, a lot of people come to visit at my dad's and my mum's and they would play games. They would play that "marrow game" it was called. Like they would take the bone of a moose and they would cook it in an open fire, then they would put it across two logs and they would blindfold each other and go round in a circle and give them an axe. And they would try to chop that bone and whoever chopped that bone, their family can eat the marrow out of the bone. But it would end up that everybody would share the marrow and they would have a lot of fun. There was a lot of laughter.

But through the drinking it all changed, eh? They didn't do that anymore unless they were drunk and when they were drunk they didn't play them games. Like they sat around, cried, listened to music or played guitar.

Now that I'm in the program and sober, and when I think of them times, you know, I thought that I was so poor but I was so rich. I had the love, the sharing, the caring my parents provided. We had the security. We had the trust.

I think about that. I think about when I was a little girl walking in the woods and I didn't know anything about the outside world 'cause we had no radio or TV. I didn't know anything about the violence. I think back to how free and safe I felt. I was a free person back there. I was born with that freedom. And in AA I got that back. I get them feelings back. I get high on life. Like I can get so high on life, a lot more higher than any drug or alcohol can get me.

It's a beautiful way of life, being able to accept who I am. I know now who I am. Like I don't have all this outside confusion where people say to me, "You know, your people are drunken Indians."

And AA has changed my attitude a lot. Like I don't feel angry anymore. I don't feel the resentment. Like I am responsible now for myself and I see that I got lost. My spirit died. It come to life through the AA program. I understand now who I am.

❧

BILL *is a fifty-two year-old Metis from Saskatchewan. A grav-el-voiced gum-chewer, his grey hair is tied in a ponytail that falls to the middle of his back. He sobered up with the help of AA five years ago and is now an addictions counsellor in a small Dene village in the Northwest Territories.*

Alcoholics Anonymous is a wonderful tool for anybody who wants to quit drinking and change their lifestyle. If they understand the terminology and the English language, eh? But our people here don't have a very strong understanding of the English language. A lot of our young people here today can't read or write grade one, two or three English.

This is a very deterring factor in relation to somebody going to treatment. They have enough understanding to go to treatment and know what's going on, but when they come and try to follow through with the aftercare of Alcoholics Anonymous meetings, the terminology is sometimes too strong for them, too far out of their reach. You try to keep the terminology as simple as possible, but it's still a difficult thing for them to relate.

AA doesn't require you to read. It doesn't require that you do anything other than sit and listen. But if you're sitting there listening to a bunch of words that you don't know what the hell they mean, eh, I would think that would be very, very frustrating, very maddening. I know it would me.

You know, when I say something to them, a simple word like "shouldn't" or "couldn't," I've had kids in here supposed to be in grade eight and they couldn't spell that word, much less know what it means.

I've promoted them to do it on their own language (*sighs*) but it just doesn't seem to take hold. I don't know what the hang-up is. I'm inclined to think that maybe because it's brought in from the outside and the attitude might be, "It's white man's program, eh? Never worked before so why is this gonna work?" I've never ever heard that, that's just a feeling I have.

RON is the forty-four-year-old Metis who was asked, as described in Chapter 10, to leave a treatment centre because the staff said he was not an alcoholic. Despite that, he has stayed sober since then and has remained active in AA. He was interviewed on a Calgary riverbank after leaving an AA meeting. He has been sober for two and a half years.

It gets very disheartening at times when you hear the same people saying the same old things at AA. There's just so much negativity. Everybody looks at the things they did when they were drinking and to me that's just like raking through the garbage. It's like keeping a bunch of old shit around and always looking at it and repeating it and saying, "This is the way we are. We're alcoholics and life is the shits and life always was the shits."

Everybody is always grasping on with their fingertips to what they've got instead of really getting out there and smelling the roses. They're looking at the thorns instead of the roses. You know, if you really want to enjoy life you got to look at the roses, smell the coffee, whatever the old catchphrases are 'cause digging through those drinking days and constantly resurrecting a way of life that's dead, for me, would be still a form of mental illness.

It's nice to have all these history books, but for Christ's sake, history's history. Let's get on with the present and the future. That's the kind of thing I enjoy — planning for the future. That's my business. I'm an engineer and I do things now that will be done next fall. I can't afford to look back to last year's projects. I'd be in a lot of trouble if I spent all my time looking back. I have to look forward.

I still go to the meetings because I know some of the people there and I enjoy the fellowship. But being around negative-thinking people bothers me. It hurts me and my growth. I'd much rather be among people who do normal things — including drinking, going to parties, going to church and living life without thoughts of addiction. But I still go to the meetings because I need to dump from time to time when I'm feeling a little hurt or a little angry or whatever.

DAVE is the thirty-one-year-old Chipewyan who, as described in Chapter 8, beat up a white man for making a joke about a "drunken squaw." He drinks only once or twice a year and then has just one or two beers. A student, he lives in a ground-floor apartment furnished in part with plastic milk cartons. He was interviewed there.

I've gone to a few AA meetings to pick up friends and I've listened to some of these stories and I think like, "Why can't you deal with this problem yourself? Why do you have to come here and tell all these people your problems?"

I think it's a wimpy way out because all my life I've dealt with my own problems. I don't go and sit in some room and cry my eyes out to some total strangers and I don't think that's the way to do it. I think you should deal with your own problems. Like, sure, if I wanted to get some advice or something, I'd go talk to one of my friends. In private. I wouldn't bring out my problem for the whole fucking world to see or hear.

Sometimes I think, "How can you sit here and tell all these people your piddly-ass problems?" Like I remember this one time going to a meeting and I heard this lady tell how her daughter told her to fuck off that day and she felt like running out and having a drink. That's a pretty lame excuse. But then I guess nobody's the same. Nobody can deal with their problems like I deal with mine. I shouldn't say anything bad about them, but I think it's just a wimpy way out.

MABEL'S STORY

Mabel is a stocky, slow-talking forty-four-year-old Kwakiutl who grew up in an Indian fishing village on the northern tip of Vancouver Island. She is an addictions counsellor and has been sober eight years.

The first time I drank I was twelve years old. It happened that my older sister and I snuck into my uncle's boat and stole a case of beer. The beer still came in tall bottles then and it tasted real sour to me. I didn't really like it, but once I took a couple of swallows, I felt a tingly feeling and I found myself really enjoying the feeling. I seem to remember drinking an awful lot. I ended up singing with my sister. I barely remember dancing with my sister in this abandoned boat that was tied up to this float. No one was around to stop us because they were all passed out.

I remember waking up feeling quite hung over. I didn't know quite what the feeling was. I just remember my mother commenting that I didn't eat breakfast. It just smelled terrible to me, although I loved my mother's cooking so much. After breakfast was over we took off across the sound to go to our old reserve. And halfway across, my stepfather stopped the boat and he called me out on deck and he shoved me overboard and he said, "You stay in the water for a while. You'll feel better when you come out."

I felt he was being really mean but it did help my hangover when I was finally pulled out of the water. And he said, "You just sit down and think about it for a while. Think about what you've done."

I remember my mum. She looked at me and gave me a kind of crooked smile and it kind of hurt that she didn't help me out or say anything.

At the age of twelve I witnessed my mother getting beaten up after a wild drinking party. They came home and there was arguing and my stepfather was quite a strong man, big man, and my mother quite sickly. I remember watching him punch her around. She was all in a heap on the floor. He hit her in the head and shortly after that she went in a coma and ended up in a hospital. She died as a result of a blood clot in her brain.

I started off a social drinker when I was about eighteen. That's when I was going with the man I married when I was nineteen. He worked for the Department of Indian Affairs, and the staff there threw a lot of parties and we'd attend. I was a social drinker and told them I didn't like the taste of it. The ladies would mix me a drink that tasted good. And then I was drinking once a week or maybe once every two weeks. I didn't really care for drinking and how I felt the next day.

My husband beat me when he was drunk and it seemed like when I knew he was gonna get mad at me, I'd drink more so I wouldn't feel the pain of his punches.

During my drinking years down on skid row in Vancouver I met a man that taught me the tricks of hustling on the street. I wasn't able to go and do my stuff while I was sober. I really felt ashamed of what I had to do to bring money in for this man and myself. So we always set aside a few dollars so I could go and get half-cut before I could go and hustle some bread. And with these few drinks in me I had the courage to play up to men and give them a good time that they were asking for. It also built up my sense of humour that I already had. My jokes flowed out freely and I didn't feel half as bad when I was out on the street.

The few times I did come home, quite a few of my relatives did try to get me to stop drinking. They tell me that I looked pretty rough and that they heard stories about me in Vancouver. I'd had quite a few close calls and they'd hear about it. They'd tell me that they were scared that the next time they heard something about me, I'd be dead. And I'd say, "Oh, no. You can't kill a good Indian," and just laugh it off.

The worst thing that happened was I didn't really care anymore. My spirit grew weak and tired and felt so useless. I had no urge to even live. I attempted suicide about four times. I slashed my wrists. One time I recall asking for a razor blade and my boyfriend gave it to me. The lady that was involved with him was at that party. I was directing my anger at her and I took it out on myself. As a result of it I ripped a nerve on my left hand and only have feeling in two of my fingers. And a great big scar. I thought the man was worth it and I thought I must really love him. In my sick mind I thought I had done the right thing and gained more of his love and respect for me. Instead I turned him off.

I never ended up in a detox centre, but I was arrested for drunkenness a total of three times. Each time I ended up in the drunk tank, I don't ever recall being put in there. I just woke up there.

Towards the end, I averaged a forty-pounder of vodka plus half a twenty-sixer a day. I can't even count how many bottles I drank. It got to the point where it tasted so good that I had to drink it faster and it was really hard for me to sip. I was ashamed of guzzling, so towards the end I drank by myself. I didn't like to drink with anyone.

I tried to quit drinking. "I won't drink when I get this welfare cheque," I'd say to myself. "I'll stay sober three days and at least I'll eat." I would always go and brag around my friends. "Gee, I haven't drank for two days now," and they'd say, "How do you do it?" And I'd say "Well, I just tell myself I don't need it." In the end I'd set myself up for another excuse to go drinking. I'd pick a fight with my boyfriend or I'd go look for trouble and say, "Aw heck, I'll just start drinking."

I made efforts to quit drinking by attending a family development centre on the west coast of Vancouver Island. My common-law husband and I and my ten-year-old son attended the treatment centre. It was a six-week session. The hardest thing about completing the treatment program was being honest with myself and letting go of friends I had made during my drinking.

I stayed sober for a total of six months. Then around Christmas time I had a slip. I drank for three months straight. After three months, I woke up one morning with the sun beating down on my body and I said, "Hey, I'm alive. I can feel the warmth. I'm sweating. There is some life in Mabel." I looked out the window and I saw blue sky and I heard a bird chirping and I said, "God! This is the day I'm gonna do it. I need Your help."

I put my feet on the floor and I walked out in the kitchen where my husband and my son were keeping quiet, 'cause they knew I'd be bitchy with a hangover. I said, "Hey, you guys, this is the day. I need your help."

I told them everything I'd require in my sobering-up, right down to keeping ice water in the fridge and putting up with my crankiness. My reward was the way they looked at me with happiness and both of them crying.

I did attend AA after that and really reached out for help and followed the steps I had learned at the treatment centre. I started building myself up spiritually, physically, emotionally and mentally.

I couldn't leave the house for a good month because I was so nervous of people looking at me or people talking to me. It took a long time to build myself up.

We lived in Richmond, B.C., and we didn't have many friends there. Most of our friends lived in Vancouver and before we went to the centre, they'd be taking a cab out to our place because they knew we had booze. After we came back, there were no more phone calls, no more visitors. But we got friends that replaced our drinking friends that came to support us. We had AA friends. We joined a support group in Richmond and there we found caring people.

After I quit drinking, I really looked at the bills I had built up, the people that I owed, and after much shame about it, I contacted these people and paid them all back. Slowly I regained self-respect in handling money. One of the things that really hurt my son was getting phone calls about NSF cheques. That really shamed him. He admitted this to me afterwards. He said, "I just want you to promise me one thing, Mum, that you never write another NSF cheque."

After being sober about a year, I got a call saying if I wanted to get a job at the treatment centre we had attended, to give them a collect call. We just ran all the way to the pay phone and called them. We waited, almost a week, and we just sat on pins and needles waiting, waiting to hear if we'd gotten a job or not, me as a daycare worker and my husband as a maintenance man. And finally we called and they said, "You're accepted. Out of eight couples that applied, you've been accepted."

We started there in 1983. We stayed there for a total of six and a half years. After four years in the daycare, I applied for the counselling job and got it. It seemed when I was in the daycare I was talking to parents and didn't realize that I was counselling.

Now that I'm sober there's one thing I know for sure — I am real. I can feel. I can taste. I can cry. I can laugh. I do so many things and really, really enjoy doing them without forcing myself. I know that I can attend a party and walk in as me without any phoneyness, without that glass of courage.

I take risks now, that's what I do different. I never used to do that before. I was scared to change. I have a new outlook on life. I sing. I play. I write poetry. And I love people. I'm relearning my language. I stumble and yet I can laugh about it without feeling ashamed. I know now that I have to feel each day for what it is and be grateful at the end of each day that I was given opportunities for change. My family tell me that I'm strong and I'm brave. My daughters tell me, "Mom, you've changed."

The best thing about sobriety is waking up alive and well. And not waking up and seeing a strange ceiling, wondering who I'm with. Not waking up with a bad-tasting mouth.

The effect that alcohol has had on me personally is a lot of losses in every area of my life. My health. My self-esteem took a while to build up. My thinking is a lot slower. Occasionally I start into stuttering. It took a while to regain use of my left hand. I've lost a few friends because I either lied to or stole from them, friends that really meant the world to me. In my sexual abuse as a child, by alcoholic men, I've built a cocoon around me. I've gained a lot of weight and haven't really tried losing it.

I have a big family and alcohol has really affected them. My grandfather and grandmother were alcoholic. My father, stepfather and my mother and all my aunts and uncles are or were alcoholics. We've drifted apart. We've become fewer in number.

A lot of deaths in my family have been alcohol-related. There's a lot of sickness now due to the heavy drinking. A lot of my cousins have given birth to FAS babies or still-born and a lot of their children have been apprehended because of alcohol. There's incest in my family due to alcohol. In one case, two children were born and I watch them suffer today because of a father and his daughter.

I've just recently moved back to the community of my family. I was away for twenty-four years. Before I left, there wasn't that much drinking going on. I'm back now and I've seen what's happened to the community. It's defaced. There's not much care for our culture. There's not very many cultural events taking place. The language is slowly dying off. We have very few elders, and the ones that we have lost have been due to alcohol.

We were raised in an isolated place where we never had electricity or things like that. We had to pack our water by hand. They took us from three isolated reserves and put us here so we could be closer to the hospital and stores instead of travelling by boat.

When they moved us here, that's when the problems started. There was still relief in them days and it was just a piece of paper saying you could get so much of groceries. We saw white people fill their shopping carts full of food, and us, we could just afford a few things. So many problems built up and pretty soon the walk to the liquor store was so inviting to go and forget.

My father was the first to die when we were moved to this community. Closer to liquor stores is what did it. There were very few houses when we came here. He didn't want to be a burden on anyone, so he decided to stay down on his friend's boat. They drank down there and he'd pass out. No bed. Just slept on the hard engine cover. Wake up. Drink. Pass out. As a result, he got double pneumonia. He died about ten days later. It was part of the reason for my leaving the community, I was so angry of what Indian Affairs had done to us.

I think differently now about native people. I used to think there was so much injustice done in putting us in residential schools, laying down laws, Indian affairs, Indian agents. And yet I've learned to turn things around and say there was some good in the residential school. That's where I learned to say, "Yes, please," and "No, thank you." That's where I learned discipline. That's where I learned how to use a knife and fork.

I sobered up for a reason. I consider myself a lighthouse for my children and my friends. I stay strong and I stay the same and let them know that I'm there for them. I shine a steady beam so that they know if ever they're in any need, that I'm there for them and whatever choices they make I'm behind them. And if they choose the wrong stream I'll always be there for them.

People come to me in my community and they ask me, "How did you do it?" I tell them straight, "It wasn't easy."

I tell them my story and they're amazed and some of them say, "I didn't know you got that bad," and I say, "I almost died from liquor."

I've helped a few people to quit drinking. Just sharing my story and not leaving any part out of it. I get a lot of teasing about being sober. I had to learn to respond in a way that leaves them thinking about what they said. And if they don't quit drinking, then I've tried to help. I don't get frustrated because I know I had a time to quit. Their time is gonna come. I'm just patient and let them know I'm still praying for them. If someone asks me, "How come you don't drink anymore?" I just tell them I don't want to die.

I curse alcohol and what it's done to me and what it's doing to my people. But if I can help anyone in any way with my story, I'll go on telling it. I've been pushed a lot to share my story but I never realized it hurts so much to tell it. I still get the urge to do myself in, but I'll talk myself up, build myself up by telling myself I'm a beautiful person. I have lots to live for. I have four grandchildren who need me. And I'm going to write stories and poems. I want to leave something behind. I went through this for a reason. And I thank God today that I'm sober and that I'm alive.

12

REASONS

"All I wanted to do was drink because of the hurt that I was feeling deep inside."

According to one study done in the mid-1980s, forty-three different academic, social, medical and government "experts" have proposed their own separate theories to explain the phenomenon of native alcoholism. None of the theories have been proven.

The theories can be grouped into three broad categories: sociological, psychological and biogenetic. One of the sociological theories says native people drink to cope with the bad feelings caused by racism. One of the psychological theories says native people are simply copying the drinking behaviours they learned from their parents who learned them, originally, from hard-drinking soldiers and fur-traders. And one of the biogenetic theories says many native people have inherited a defective gene that causes them to become alcoholic. (The premise under which Alcoholics Anonymous operates, that alcoholism is a disease, falls within the biogenetic category.) Some of the theories fall strictly within one category, but most are combinations that borrow bits and pieces from several categories.

A 1984 survey of native addictions counsellors in Saskatchewan listed eight reasons to explain native alcoholism. The reason listed most often was the loss of cultural identity; followed by poverty and unemployment.

The various experts aside, however, the ones most affected by the problem — native people themselves — have their own explanations.

THREEBEAR *is a quiet, muscular and athletic thirty-one-year-old Blood from southern Alberta. He was interviewed in a native treatment centre. He has been sober for twenty-eight days.*

I was brought up in a good family. My parents never drank. My old man is a medicine man. My uncle is a medicine man. So I grew up around all that. But I never had the guidance. My mother was always bus driving. My dad was always gone and I was always home alone. It's just that I never had the guidance while I was growing up. I think that's where my drinking problem started, I just needed guidance.

LAZARUS *is the husky, smiling seventy-four-year-old Stoney elder who said, in Chapter 1, that the word for alcohol in his language meant "crazywater."*

There must be something in the blood of the Indian. You see the white people, they can drink but they'll be more careful than the Indians. They'll know how much they're taking and they'll realize that they should stop right there. That's the intention that the white people have. But with the Indians, they'll never stop until they're out.

There's no difference between the white people's blood and Indian blood, or Indians' brain and white man's brain and so on. But I always think there must be something because look at the white people. They don't get mad. Oh, maybe some of them do, eh? But look at the white people. They have a social drink, a man and wife, they are so lovingly each other. They enjoy drinking and they take off and they go to bed without causing any trouble. But when an Indian start to drink they start to fight with his wife or her husband and they go different ways.

I don't know, there must be something in the blood.

BETTY *is a no-nonsense, chain-smoking forty-one-year-old Metis. She had a traditional upbringing on a trapline in northern Alberta, and is now a social counsellor. She was interviewed in the basement of a community service organization in Edmonton.*

I was really raised a native way. They didn't teach us English and they raised us in the bush. They taught us that you need to be tough. They told us that you can never show the white man that you're weak. They show their weakness in tears and you can't do that. If you cried, then you were a weak person. You need to be strong. You need to (*sighs*) not cry. Like you're weak if you cry.

So when we were hurt when we were kids, we would go away in the bush and we'd cry by ourselves. We would not allow our brothers and sisters along to go and cry too. We were raised that way. I never showed any emotions. I just sort of acted tough. I was a good pretender. I'd pretend that everything was okay when it wasn't.

When I went to school I just would not communicate with any teachers. We were told not to share anything about the things that happened at our home. My dad was a medicine man. Things that happened in our house, we were not able to share with them — our sweetgrass, any of our native ways — we were not allowed to discuss in school or with our friends. That was just something that was sacred around our home.

So when I came to the city, I began to realize that I was different and people began to discriminate me and call me a "squaw," "lazy bum," "drunk" and all these things. I really resented white people because of that. I would not trust them. I didn't want any white person near me. Down the drag there was native people there. I felt good. I felt free. I felt I was accepted and could be trusted. But there was a lot of anger, a lot of hurt. I just suppressed all the feelings and I just drank. I used alcohol as an escape.

MARK is the hulking, tough-talking forty-six-year-old Mohawk who said, in Chapter 10, that people who work in native treatment centres should not be paid. He has been sober for twenty years.

I hear a lot of kids say they drink because they want to *belong*. The white man uses that word "peer pressure." I think that's bullshit. They do it because *they want to*.

You can blame the governments of the United States and Canada for introducing the alcohol. But you also got to blame our people for *accepting* it. They didn't have to accept it. They didn't have to indulge in that stuff.

A lot of people want to blame other things for what they do and that's wrong, 'cause that's *you*. *You're* the one that's goin' into that bar and puttin' your money down and pickin' that bottle up. *You're* doin' it. Tryin' to blame something or someone is a cop-out.

MAGGIE is a forty-six-year-old Carrier, originally from British Columbia. She is the executive director of a native-run training centre for addictions workers in Alberta and has been a leader in the field of native addictions for more than twelve years. She was interviewed between sessions of a native addictions conference in an Edmonton hotel.

I believe that the drinking stems from a loss of sense of self, which happened with the outlawing of ceremony a hundred years ago. Ceremony brought meaning to life — ceremonies for birth; ceremonies when girls had their first menstruation and became a woman and her body was something to be honoured; ceremonies when young boys became men; ceremonies based on names; ceremonies dealing with death and pain.

Now we have a high death rate and no vehicle in which to deal with that pain. And the outlawing of ceremony was done just before the really big push for residential school. The whole structure of relationships within the community was devastated with that first law outlawing ceremonies and with residential school.

I think that three groups were responsible. The biggest influence at that time was the churches. The churches had a vested interest to Christianize the Indian community and that wasn't possible when the ceremonies were in place. The second group that was responsible was the Canadian government, because they allowed that law to pass. And the third group was the Canadian population, because they thought it was acceptable. They misunderstood Indian ceremony as being superstition, and people weren't being properly assimilated if they were still involved in ceremony. They didn't understand that ceremony had tied to it the value of life, the value of self, the value of spirit.

The other thing is that our people never learned a process of drinking which is common, say, in France, where it's been there thousands of years. The people who traded liquor to them actively encouraged them to become intoxicated because it effected a cheaper sale of their goods. And then when people were not allowed to drink in licensed facilities, that set up a process in which people tended to gulp their drinks, so it was another socialization of an alcoholic drinking process.

The other thing that contributed to it was a massive amount of unresolved pain from the loss of relationship and a tremendous amount of abuse that people experienced in residential school and in their communities.

And there has been a continuation of the violence and the high death rate. In many communities the ceremonies were not intact to deal with that unresolved grief. So you just start piling pain on pain.

ROBERT is a twenty-five-year-old Indian from a small village in northern Canada. Handsome and fashionably dressed, he is effeminate and speaks with a slight stutter. He was interviewed in a native treatment centre.

One of the reasons I started drinking was because I had been sexually abused. I came to in the nursing station. I tried my best to try to tell them, but it wouldn't come out. It just stayed there. They kept bugging me and bugging me and I couldn't bring it out. I just told them, "I want to go home." After I got home my mum and dad were passed out, so I just locked the door. I was just a small child at that time. I was only twelve years old. That really hurted me a lot.

I started drinking when I was twelve and I quit until I was about fifteen. I got sexually abused again, that's when I really started to drink. I didn't care anymore. The second time I got sexually abused I left my home town. I didn't want anybody to know about it and I stayed away for a long, long time. I really started to drink. I'd drink every chance I had. I used to go to parties every single night. I never go to school. All I wanted to do was drink because of the hurt that I was feeling deep inside.

And the third time, the time that I *really* started to drink, I'd been at this one party and the same person was there that sexually abused me when I was twelve. He waited till everybody was drunk and he did the same thing to me again. I tried to fight back. The third time he sexually abused me, I was torned up all inside. I had stitches all inside. But still yet I wouldn't come out and say who did it to me.

I keep holding it deep inside and every time I drank I would get in a fight, get in an argument with anybody that was around me. And the violence that I did to other people — I tried killing them, I tried stabbing them, I tried shooting them. I tried every which way to get that feeling off my chest because I felt so dirty inside.

I started to commit suicide. About five times. The first time I shot my left foot. I was drunk at that time and I was falling around and that gun just went off and it hit my foot. I meant to shoot my head. My foot didn't heal because I was drinking too much. I had to get my foot cut off 'cause it got infected and it was going green, eh? So they had to cut it off.

Anyways, as years went by I attended school in town. I used to get in fights with other students. I go to school, lunchtime I go home. I'd have a bottle in my room, I'd take a couple shots. I feel better and then I go back to school in the afternoon. After school I would go downtown and go straight into the bars and not go home sometimes two, three days. I went on and on like that for at least eight months.

After a while I realized that I had a problem and so I decided I better go back to my home town. So I quit school, went back home. When I went back home my sisters started to drink a lot. We started to get in fights. The whole family was getting into fights. I stab a person but I never killed a person. I just slashed their arm. One day I was really mad and I went out drinking and I got in a fight with this one lady and after I went home, I grab a gun, a thirty-thirty. I load it up. My mum and dad was standing to me, begging me, crying to me and telling me not to do that to myself. I shot in the air twice. I didn't know what I was doing. I'd been drinking quite a lot.

I was standing by the kitchen table with a thirty-thirty and two cops walked in and asked me to put the gun down. They were pointing guns at me too and I didn't care if they shot me or if I shot myself because I was in a state where I was ready to commit suicide. Anyways, I just put that gun down and I started to cry.

The next morning I looked around and I realized I was in jail. The cop opened the cell and he asked me if I knew what happened last night and I told him, "No." He explained that I had a gun and was bound to commit suicide. And I thought to myself right there that I really do have a drinking problem. I have to make a commitment to take treatment to do something for myself, to become a better person.

After I left the jail, I went home and I made arrangements to go to treatment. And now to this day, I've been sober one year, ten months and a half. My drinking problem has been pretty well under control and now I'm attending Poundmaker's to deal with the sexual abuse. (*sighs*) Sometimes it's hard to bring out stuff that I don't want to, but I make myself because I want to get it off my chest and just have nothing to do with it anymore. I want to be free from it.

I haven't talked about it with anybody before until I came here. And it's helping me so far. It's helping me a lot. I was a shy person and now I can talk in front of anyone.

After I get back home I'm gonna confront this person and tell him what my plans is. The first guy who sexually abused me passed away six years. But this other person, I'm going to confront him and take him to court. It's never too late to bring it up again. I'm not scared anymore.

EVERETT'S STORY

Everett is forty-six years old with brooding eyes, a dark scowl and a cutting sense of humour. He is confined to a wheelchair in his home on the Blood reserve in southern Alberta. Everett was a well-known cartoonist and reporter before sobering up eight years ago.

I was born with muscular dystrophy, and when I was a teenager I injured my shoulder and I began to waste away on my arm. Then I injured my pelvic area and the muscles began to waste away in the girdle area. And then I broke my left arm and the muscles began to waste away to where they were just skin and bones.

I used to wear short sleeves in the summer and people began to look at me funny. People began to gossip, "What's wrong with him?" The doctors said it was incurable and I thought I was going to die fairly soon because most people did not know very much about muscular dystrophy back then.

A lot of times I was taken for a retarded person 'cause I'm hard of hearing, which makes me look even more stupid. So it all began to create a lot of problems for me. I became very reclusive for about four years and I never really associated with anybody. I spent all my time in the pool hall setting pins and playing pool upstairs out of sight of everybody.

I had this horrible, horrible image of myself as a disabled person. I began to think of myself as some freak and monster and it just gnawed away at me on the inside. Although I had physical deformities, it's nothing compared to the wart that was created in my mind.

When I was twenty-one, I left home and went to school in Banff to study art. I drank with the other students and I think I drank very sociably. There was no hangover, no nothing. It was limited to a few glasses and that was all. Towards the end, a cousin who was living in Calgary started coming to visit on weekends. That was when I began to drink heavy.

Drinking made me a very sociable person. It enabled me to do a lot of things. When I drank I became Mr. Hyde. Dr. Jekyll was forgotten and then I became Mr. Hyde and I had a marvellous time. It gave me a chance to loosen my tongue. Eventually it got too loosened and I think I became the most obnoxious person in the world. I was always shooting off my mouth.

I was always terribly afraid to approach girls. That was one of the things that I liked about drinking because I could approach a girl. I never really knew them other than these bar hoppers, you know, mostly Indian girls. Back home, in Cardston, you don't look at white women, you know. These are Mormons, the pure white race, and you just don't mix with them.

That town has a lot to do with my attitude towards white people. At a very early age I was conditioned that Indians were second class. I was always treated as an inferior and to make things worse, my people treated me as an inferior because of being disabled.

Nobody has ever written about the discrimination within Indian reserves. That's where it hurts most. Not by a damn white person. White person is a stranger. Tell him to fuck off. They can treat you any damn way, it's not going to bother you 'cause you don't know the person. But when somebody you know slights you, that hurts. That's where the damn sickness is in ourselves, the way we treat each other.

Indian people looked on my disability as a curse — that I did something very wicked and it was a punishment. A lot of Christian people told me that God is punishing me for the wrong I did, the evil that was in my mind, in my heart. I thought, "Damn it. Am I that terrible? Hitler must be a lot better because he was a hell of a lot healthier than I am."

I became repulsed by religion because of their condemning preachings. I turned to atheism and agnostic teachings. I claimed to be an atheist because I was really mad and angry at religion because they could not help. I even went to the cults, but I was quickly turned off because they would tell me that I was a disabled person because I was a very wicked person in my *last* life.

The greatest drinking problem I had was in the years '68 to '82, which were exactly the years I was working with *Kainai News*. As a cartoonist and as a reporter, it was an occupational hazard. For one thing, there was plenty of it flowing around. I covered a lot of political meetings and the booze flowed freely and a lot of people bought me drinks so I wouldn't draw cartoons of them, but that didn't save them.

In the years I was working I was drinking almost every day. Every time I go to Calgary, Edmonton or anywhere, I got drunk. I never planned it that way, it just happened. The liquor was flowing and I drank. Pretty soon I became more and more dependent on it. I had to have a little snort to get me going. I had to have a mid-day lift. I needed an eye-opener. I needed a nightcap. I needed it all the time. I really became very dependent on alcohol. And meanwhile it was destroying my life.

Just before I quit, it almost killed me. I was bleeding for about six weeks, my liver was all damaged and the doctor told me, "You have a choice — to live or to die."

I knew I had muscular dystrophy. I knew I was not going to live that long but that's not what was bothering me. What was bothering me was I was more afraid of becoming a vegetable.

I don't want to blame *Kainai News*. I don't want to blame anybody. All my drinking was a result of my inability to cope with my disability. I quit in '82 because *Kainai News* kind of forced me to quit. My superiors told me that I was gonna be in the gutters. That really woke me up because it was true. I was gonna be in the gutters and all I was gonna be was nothing but a damn drunk. Before that, at least I had some social standing. I made money. I had some recognition and whatnot, but I realized that without a job I am an absolute bum.

I never went to a treatment centre myself. I just more or less quit on my own. I sobered up eight years ago, but each day I feel as though I only sobered up last week or the day before.

Today I have a lot of problems with being disabled. I'm practically incarcerated at home. I have a great deal of trouble moving around. Only when my brother is here am I able to go out and socialize a bit. It's extremely difficult and I know that my health is getting worse. I'm going to be confined to a bed fairly soon and I thought being incarcerated in a home was bad enough but now I'm beginning to realize that, *dammit*, in the very near future I'm going to be imprisoned in my mind, in a body that is going to be damn useless. All I'm going to have is my mind and what the hell am I going to do?

I think I can cope now with just having a mind. I'm not too worried about it. I'm expecting it and it's not bothering me terribly. This is what made me turn to spiritual help. With the help of a lot of people, I began going back to church. I'm still not really a churchgoer but I go to church occasionally. I read the Bible daily as some sort of spiritual help.

I have a terrible guilt that's in me because I believe I killed a lot of people and one of them was my kid brother. I introduced alcohol to him and he died in a car accident on his way to get a drink with his friends. I take that blame and it really is devastating. I had a cousin who was dying of diabetes. I continually supplied liquor to him because I felt sorry for him and because I was drinking and that killed him too. I had an uncle, again, the same thing. I knew alcohol was going to kill and I kept supplying him. And you start thinking back, "*Dammit*. You are a responsible person. Why the hell are you doing such irresponsible things like getting people drunk? Especially younger people?"

I'm not an alcohol counsellor, but I'd do everything I can to discourage other people now because I see it's absolutely no damn good. Yet some people try to justify social drinking. They always say *ah-sooks-su-mee* — somebody that drinks good, sociable drinker, it means drinking good. But I see absolutely no good.

Some people say it relaxes you and all that. But there are other things that are just as good. Sex. Food. You name it. There's a lot of other things you can do that can be relaxing.

I've been able to stay off drinking. It's kind of funny, I wanted to drink to socialize, but since I quit I'd just as soon enjoy myself. I find a lot of pleasure in solitude. It gives me a chance to write. It gives me a chance to do my artwork. I have a lot more interests than I used to — my artwork, sculpture, painting. It keeps me busy all day long. It's a nice pastime. I'm doing them very slowly, but at least I'm doing them.

I'm on a short income that's just keeping me alive and there's not a heck of a lot for luxury. But the luxury now is I'm able to have time. For the first time I'm listening to music and appreciating it. Before it was just background, you know, just blasting away and I never really paid any attention to it. Now I listen to all kinds of music. I have a greater appreciation for the beauty around me. Like it's a nice day today. It's the simplest things that are the greatest gifts. I'm thankful I have friends that have stuck with me throughout all these years.

I do a lot more reading. I'm working as a volunteer with the hospital in Lethbridge. I've done volunteer work with the young offenders. I taught in jail with inmates there. I'm on the advisory committee for native adult education. I've taught cartooning. I'm involved with disabled groups. I'm involved with the premier's council on persons with disabilities. And for the first time I'm trying to really contribute. I'm trying to help other disabled people to quit drinking.

I got a lot of recognition as a cartoonist and as somebody who was doing great things for his people. I kind of think that was a damn lie. I wasn't doing a damn thing. I was just saying the obvious. I was saying cliches. Altruistic bullshit, that's all it was. Besides that, most of the stories were stolen from the bar. I went and bought drinks for these people and they told me the stories and I put it in the *Kainai News*.

I was terribly frustrated. I wanted to quit, but I kept drinking. I was getting suicidal. I tried committing suicide about three different occasions. And the alcohol, all it did was make the problems worse and worse. I never wanted to face my life. I don't think I was really alive. I was just going through the motions and I didn't care. But now that I do, nobody's around me. I'm a hell of a lonely person now. I'm not saying I'm *lonely*. I'm just saying nobody's around. I don't get any visitors. I only get visitors like you and anthropologists and historians that come around and ask questions. That's good company to me.

Now I look back at the fourteen years where I really drank heavy. I think there was a heck of a lot I could have done but I didn't do it. I think that's the greatest harm I ever did. Drinking was a waste of time. It's a bloody waste of time. Money, I don't miss. But I miss the things I wish I could have done.

I always thought when I got on a wheelchair I would kill myself because it's too degrading. That was a source of comfort to me, "When I'm on a wheelchair, I'm gonna kill myself." I was feeling bad 'cause I knew I was not going to be able to walk. So what did I do? I drank and staggered around. (*laughs*) And then when I got on a wheelchair, I quit drinking!

But when I got there, it wasn't so bad. As a matter of fact I feel I've accomplished a heck of a lot more since I got on a wheelchair. And inside I'm more serene. I feel a lot better about myself and I'm doing a lot of things that make me feel good.

I have absolutely no inclination now to drink. That's not part of my life. If somebody wants to do it, that's their business. I will try to discourage them if I can, but most of the time it's too much of a hassle because at first they'll joke with you and then they'll gradually start picking on you, ridiculing you and bad-lipping you. So it's just for practical purposes that I don't associate with people that drink. And they never make sense. By George! There's nothing more boring in the world than a friendly drunk. They're terribly boring, they're repetitious. I can't stand a drunk because a lot of times they remind me of me. You know, and here I thought I had something important to say when I was drinking! I thought I was *saying* something.

When I first sobered up I tried to avoid drunken Indians. Now I accept them. I'm not ashamed of it. Like people say they are very ashamed when they see an Indian is drinking. But what about the way council rips off the people? What about the people in the administration or the elite of the reserve, the way they ripped off the poor? Isn't that even worse than somebody drinking?

It's terribly degrading to be unemployed, to crawl up to social service and welfare and unemployment and try to get your cheque. They'll drag you through the fucking shit all the time. It's damn disgusting. I know disabled people who refuse to go to welfare. They'd sooner just bum off the street and drink. I hate to see these disabled people drinking and I see a lot of them drinking because they can't cope with their disability. I'm hoping to reach some other disabled people because my drinking problem had more to do with being disabled than being a native.

13

SOLUTIONS

"You gotta make them want to be Indian. You gotta have their heart belong to them again as warriors — not as a bunch of scavenging idiots that this society created."

What should be done to "solve" the native alcoholism "problem"? Is the sobriety-based treatment philosophy of Alcoholics Anonymous the answer? Or should social drinking be promoted as an alternative, especially for young people? Given that some people blame native alcoholism on social, economic or biogenetic causes, what role should government or the medical community play? And what part should traditional native healing practises or spiritual beliefs play in the treatment process? Should alcohol be banned in native communities? Should addictions workers and native community leaders be required to be non-drinkers?

These are the kinds of questions posed by the present situation. With few exceptions, there is no consensus. In the native community, however, there is almost unanimous agreement that any "solution" will have to be based on two fundamental points:

• Progress must be made on self-government, land claims and economic development; and

• There must be a cultural and spiritual revival in the native community.

MARY is a thin, soft-spoken fifty-two-year-old Cree from a reserve in northern Manitoba.

When I pray at night, I ask God to help me to have a dry reserve. It would be much better. I still think that every day. I want a dry reserve because there's lot of trouble going on, eh? Sometimes they beat up someone and they break the windows. That's what they do, eh? Them drunkards does that. They shoot. With a gun.

My boy got shot last year with a shotgun. He's twenty-four. He got shot on the leg 'cause them boys didn't like him. That's why. That's what they do when they drink. They fight each other 'cause they're jealous.

He was sleeping and I heard somebody push the door open. Six of them. They're from up the hill over there. And a boy said, "Where's David?"

I told him David is sleeping and they went in the room right away and wake him up. They all grabbed him off the bed. Start fighting. They throw full bottles of beer inside the house. Broke them. And there was sick kids inside the house, even little babies. He went out and those boys went and shoot him on the leg.

So I phoned the cops. The cops came right away, they took that guy to jail, that one that shot my boy in the leg. He's okay now.

It happens a lot around here. That's why I'm wishing for a dry reserve.

MAGGIE is a forty-six-year-old Carrier. She is the executive director of a native-run training centre for addictions workers. She has been a leader in the field of native addictions for more than twelve years.

I don't believe that alcohol should be outlawed but I also don't believe that we should have liquor stores or bars in our communities because there are many people who would not consume substances if it wasn't readily available.

There are some people who'll go to a bootlegger, but their wives often wouldn't consume or their children wouldn't consume. But if it becomes something where they can go across the street, then they would. So I think that the danger of inviting people who aren't presently substance abusers into that process is much higher if you have that outlet real close.

Alkali Lake does not have a prohibition policy. Never has had. They have a form of social pressure which says, "If you want to be an active member of this community, it's important that you be an abstainer. If you are a substance abuser, we'll do everything we can to assist you to get help."

These people don't say, "You can't come to the dance." They don't say, "You can't consume it." They just say, "If you're gonna come to this activity, the sober dance, this potluck supper, it's important you not be consuming alcohol. You're not going to be socially acceptable."

LOUISE is a middle-aged addictions worker on an Alberta reserve. She has been sober for fourteen years.

The cycle that we're in has to be broken somehow and that starts with the kids. Not to preach, "Don't drink. Don't drink." But to teach them even if their parents are drinking, they don't have to. Preaching, "Don't drink, drinking is bad," is bad as far as I can see. Maybe we should teach the kids that there is such a thing as responsible drinking, if there is such a thing. It's okay to drink a beer here or there, but don't get drunk on it. And that goes contrary to my job as a prevention worker.

I don't think alcohol should be banned entirely on reserves. Prohibition just makes it that much more attractive. Instead of banning it, it might be better to expose children to responsible drinking, instead of total abstinence.

BARBARA is the director of a native treatment centre in northern Canada.

All my staff have to be sober for several years before they can even work here. There would be problems if I hired a social drinker or if I allowed my staff to work here as counsellors if they continued to be social drinkers. Because as staff members we have to set a good example for the community.

This is a brand-new treatment centre. There's a lot of people in this community that drink. If they see that a lot more Indian people are becoming sober, then they will make an effort to enter our treatment facility. They would question if our staff drank and they seen them drinking. Word gets around pretty fast. "Why is that person working here when they're drinking? What kind of a treatment facility is that? Why don't they practise what they preach?" is what they'd say.

We also don't encourage our clients to be social drinkers. We try to help them on their road to recovery and to stop drinking altogether. In our feasibility study, it was found that there were about five generations of alcoholics in the North. These people have grown up generation after generation in alcoholic homes. How do you think they could be social drinkers? A lot of these people are chronic alcoholics and have been drinking for many years. You can see it from their face. When they drink, they will drink for weeks. So you tell me how they can possibly be social drinkers? They are beyond that.

ELANA is a short and chunky thirty-seven-year-old Blood. She was interviewed at Stoney Medicine Lodge, a native treatment centre in southern Alberta.

Role models are really important to any community and it really does make a lot of difference. The councillor here, Rose, is from my reserve and she has helped so many on our reserve to recover because they see her and they say, "I can do that." They know how she was when she was an alcoholic and I know a lot of people have really tried hard on account of Rose. They say, "If she can do it, I can do it too."

I admire her too and I use her as my role model now.

And that's exactly what I'm thinking now, "If Rose can do it, I can too."

WALTER *is a tough-looking thirty-six-year-old Cree-Assiniboine from Saskatchewan. He was interviewed on the edge of Calgary's skid row while he waited to be admitted to a public treatment centre. He has been sober for eighteen days.*

I didn't have an older brother. I didn't have a role model to look up to. I was shipped around from one foster home to the next and pretty well had to fight my own battles. That's how I became addicted, trying to drown my problems and be somebody that I really wasn't.

I think role models, definitely, they make an impression on a youngster that's starting to go astray. Especially nowadays. They need someone that they can say, "Hey, I wanna be just like him when I grow up."

I know that, because my little nephew sees me as one of those people, eh? He sees me as going to university and somebody that's always working and he doesn't see the drunken side of me. He sees me having drinks, but he's usually in bed before I get drunk. So I try my best not to get drunk in front of him, eh? And he says, "Uncle Walter's the best," eh?

Yeah, role models are definitely a must for native children.

JOSEPHINE *is a shrivelled but forthright seventy-six-year-old Blood. She was interviewed in her home on the Blood reserve in southern Alberta.*

I don't think there's anybody that can do anything about it because the only one that's going to help you is yourself. And if you turn to God. That's the only solution.

Make up your mind. Have the determination that you're going to quit and turn to God for help and I'm sure He'll hear you and He will help you. It's the only solution. There's no help you can turn to, not the alcoholic treatments or anybody. Yourself alone is the one to help you. And turn to God.

JER'S STORY

Jer is a fast-talking forty-two-year-old Ojibway from northern Ontario. Tall and skinny with long hair, his speech is punctuated with dramatic gestures and comic expressions. A house painter and part-time dope-dealer, he quit drinking two days ago. He was interviewed in a Vancouver hotel room.

Let's start from the beginning. Born winter '49, trapping shack, northern Ontario. Delivered by my older sister. Mum died of tuberculosis three months after giving me birth. Dad died a year and a half later. I was raised by my grandfather, my oldest brother — he was fourteen years older than me — and a succession of aunts and uncles.

At the age of eight one fall, I was in a little community called Collins and I'd heard talk of my cousins going to a place called "school." They all jumped on a train one day, this passenger train that happened to be sittin' there all night. I was on that train, playing. We were running up and down the cars and the next thing you know, the train moved. I wasn't supposed to be on there, but I wanted to see where this train went. Being in a community where it's all native and everybody knows each other, nobody was actually my guardian, so nobody thought it was different that I was on this train.

When I got to the residential school in Sioux Lookout, they realized I had no business being there. They figured I was just an abandoned person, (*laughs*) so they told me I could be a student. I was with a few cousins, so I said that was all right, this was fun.

Next came the school part. I didn't know how to speak English. They asked me my name. I gave them my name. They hit me. They asked me again what my name was. I gave them my name, they hit me again.

I didn't know this then, but I was being beaten for speaking my language. So finally a woman teacher hit me with a stick and then I took the stick, I broke the stick. I took a book and threw it at her. I hit her. Right in the face. From then on I was in trouble.

They sent me to another school in Kenora. It was kind of like a reform school. I was only a nine-year-old kid then. I was there for a year and they sent me back to the school in Sioux Lookout. After Sioux Lookout, they sent me to residential school in Sault Ste. Marie. In that school, there was always fights, there was always anguish. There was people running away from there. We were at each other's throats.

There was a lot of deaths in those schools, a real lot. I know names of people that died in those schools, their parents didn't even know what happened to them. There's children running around in the bush in northern Quebec and Ontario, illegitimate children of the priests that used to rape the girls in school.

I graduated at eighteen. That's ten years to get through twelve years of school. I don't find that exceptional. I just got tired of being hit. (*laughs*) You either learn or get hit. One or the other.

In 1967 I graduated out of grade twelve and I went home 'cause my brother was murdered then. Over booze, by his best friend, his best friend for all his life. They were drinking. I never had a chance to sit down and have a legitimate beer with him. I went to school and graduated, just so he could be proud of me 'cause he was the only parent I had. And I went home to bury him the year I graduated. Fuck. What a way to live.

There's 120 miles of track between Sioux Lookout and Armstrong. Our people live in all these communities in between. When you live on a railroad line, the train brings you your boxes of beer and the groceries and whatever else. But there's never just groceries. Never. Sometimes cases of whiskey. For every case that they unload, they're also unloading coffins. It's like they're unloading coffins instead of boxes of beer.

From the time my brother was murdered, that's when I really tied into the beer. I crawled into the bottle after that. I worked on the railroad and I started boozing heavily. Then I got sick of that scene and I just wanted to get the hell away. So I came to B.C. I went to college here in Vancouver and I did every imaginable drug here. I banged up for two years on MDA. I was on mescaline, heroin, opium, pot, acid, you name it. Then I started hangin' around with junkies. I started watching them squabble about it. Jesus jumpin', they would tear each other apart and I said, "These guys are supposed to be friends?"

I knew there was something wrong, and I knew if I stayed here I'd become a junkie and die, so I left and went to Prince Rupert to work in a pulp mill. But Prince Rupert (*laughs*) aah, what a place to go. I go from a junkie to a boozehound because Prince Rupert, the sun never shines, it rains constantly. I mean, where you gonna go? You can't go outside for a walk, or play ball. All there was doing up there was the bars and that's where *everybody* went. There was no other place *to* go. So we all went to the bar. At least I got off the junk. I sure got into the booze, though. Holy shit.

So when I was working there I went to dealing dope. Made a lot of money at it. But the law got kind of hot there, so I split and went back to Ontario and I went to work in the mines. I made tons of money again and drank tons and tons of beer again. Then I got fired from there because of booze. Jesus. So I went down the road and got hired at another mine. Quit there because I was too damn drunk to go back to work. I started realizing what booze was doing to me, so I quit the mines. I went to Edmonton and worked there during the oil boom. It wasn't long before I was goin' from town to town to town.

In Winnipeg I was charged with attempted murder and yet the guy tried to murder me. He knocked me down and he sat on my chest. The *son of a bitch*. He weighed *310 pounds* and me weighing 140. The guy's sitting on me and he's punching my head. I found this little shank and I hit him with it. I had no choice. He didn't even *feel* it and he wouldn't move. Then he started looking for that damn wine bottle to pound me with. I shafted him again and then I shoved him off of me. I called the damn ambulance for the son of a bitch or else he would'a *died*. But, no, they charged *me* with attempted murder 'cause I stabbed him twice. They said, "You should have stabbed him only once." And they wonder why we drink.

I pled guilty to wounding with intent to maim and disfigure. I took out his spleen and a couple other things. (*laughs*) I got two years' probation, and the day I was free from that I came back to Vancouver.

When I moved out here, I ran into Terry and she was just a barfly, but she was fun. We used to scrounge around together and find ten dollars so we could buy a gram of pot and go sit in the bar and see who would buy us a beer.

Now we have two children. Six years later, she's taking me to court for assault. I did not assault her. I did slap her the week before for some stupid move of hers. I'll admit to that, but this one, she charged me and she couldn't retract it because the law changed so that you can't pull out.

There's a few things you have to understand. I'm a life skills coach. I've worked for a lot of native organizations. I'm not an idiot. I might be a boozer and I've done a few things that are not exactly kosher, but I know one thing — if talking don't work, a good one upside the head does make a big difference. It might not work altogether, but you sure get the person's attention.

She used to smoke pot. We used to have the grandest times. And from the time she was pregnant, she quit. (*snaps his fingers*) Like that. But she quit the pot and went to the booze. Some *asshole* told her that pot was worse for her than booze was. Yeah. And all the way through both of her pregnancies she drank. I told the hospitals, the police, the so-called native counsellors, the AA counsellors. You think any of them did a damn thing? *Fuck no*. I end up in jail.

So now I happen to be serving a year and a half probation and all I was doing was preventing her from breastfeeding my son. We were drinking. I was trying to pull my kid away because she'd been drinking for four hours. She didn't eat nothing. And I know that whatever goes in her mouth goes into her tit if you're breastfeeding and she was literally feeding that kid *booze*. Alcohol shake. I went to court and yet the law wouldn't do nothing about it. They convicted *me* of assault.

I live over here because it's too fucking cold at home and if I go back to Ontario I know my lifespan ain't gonna be very long. Not in northern Ontario. I've been running away because there's nowhere I belong anyway. I got no reserve. We never signed a treaty. We were the rogue band that wandered around northwestern Ontario and never got a reserve. We belong to bands but we never lived on those bands. Like Fort Hope is mine. I've never lived there. I've got no house there. Those people over there don't know who I am. Some of my family's there, from *way* back, hundreds of years ago. But you're fucking crazy you think I'm gonna live way the hell up four hundred miles north in the middle of *nowhere*. Can you see me up there?

What is there to go home to? What's everybody at home doing now? I mean this cold night? *They're boozing.* We could sit around and drink coffee all damn night, but not for very long. We could make snowshoes, but for what? We don't have to chase animals in the deep snow to make a living anymore 'cause there's no more trapping. There's nowhere up there to live. There's nothing to *do*. You can only cut so much wood. You can only fish so much fish and you can only hunt so many animals. It only takes up so much time. We got no cars. We got no sidewalk. We got no store down the corner. We got no pavement. We got no nothing. We got no electricity. We got no *nothing* at home.

So you're bored up there. What do you do? You go back down to the city. First thing on the agenda, "Let's go get a bottle. Cheaper than a bootlegger at home. Let's get four or five bottles."

I ask these people here, "Why do you live in the city?"

"I got no house on the reserve, man."

Well, if you live your life the real true way, the way it is supposed to be, you have enough friends who respect you enough to help you build your own house. You don't need the government. You know what I mean? But that's all I hear, "Oh, they haven't built my house."

They waiting for *somebody else* to do their thing. *And they're sitting down here sucking on the fucking bottle.* Why can't they get the initiative together and build their own house? You'd find a lot of people, if they had to do that, they wouldn't have time to sit in the bars and booze. That's true. You wouldn't have the time. They'd build something. They'd create. It seems that the native's creatability is gone, is taken away through booze.

Booze has got me nothing in all my life but trouble. Every instance in my life there has been a malfunction, it's come through booze. I went to jail on booze. My brother was murdered on booze. My separation from my wives has been on booze. My oldest son ran away from his mother because of booze. Most of my relatives are dead because of booze. I've hurt the people I love the most on booze.

But I don't find nothing really wrong with alcohol, shy that it's too accessible and it should not be allowed on reserves at all. If people bootleg on reserve, they should be banned from that reserve for a period of five years. And don't ban just the person that's doing this shit, ban the whole family.

"You, son, you're the bad guy. Take your dad and get out of here. *Yeah, go on. You don't have enough sense to raise your kids properly, get off there too. We don't need you.* Look what you raised your kids at. What fuckin' good are you to us now?"

You know?

Natives used to do this before. This is nothing new. This used to happen hundreds of years before the white man ever came. We banished people.

"*You wanna shit around with this community? You wanna fuck around with it?* Okay. We're not about to take it. *You* take *your* family and you go fuck them *white* people around. Let's see how good you are at fucking them people around."

My life has been mine because of some very tragic circumstances. But all these other people that got trapped in the residential school system, like I did, they are all dead. They stayed home. They never learned how to speak English very well by which they could get employment and improve their lifestyle or whatever. They stayed at home and they drank at home. And they *murdered* each other at home. And they died by other means — drowning and freezing to death. But those people were intoxicated when they died in their skidoos and their boats on those open lakes by their judgments being fucked up by booze.

My cousin Julie, a couple of years ago I phoned her up and I asked her about the young men my age, my cousins and whatnot. There used to be twenty-five or thirty of us that always used to hang around together. We were in our early twenties, just young bucks, happy and we knew what to do with a hard-on. Anyway, I phoned up Julie and she says none of them are left. They're all dead. All of them. They're all gone.

I can bitch about the life that I was dealt, the cards I was dealt in my life, but if I was not dealt those cards, I could be dead too, 'cause I would have been partying and drinking up and getting mad and fisticuffing around until I was shot.

Anyway, I tried to prove my worth to this society and to my people as a successful man that went out and did this and this. I pushed my ass, man. I pushed myself to the limit. I graduated out of grade twelve. I pushed myself so I got a mechanic's ticket. I pushed myself in heavy-duty mechanics. And I pushed myself all the way until I got everything. And then when I did have everything, a nice pick-up truck, a nice home, got this and that and thousands of dollars, *where's the respect, boys, where's the respect?*

I partied with white people but I started realizing something. On the job, when they needed my help I was their greatest buddy. When I came down to the urban centres, "Oh, Jer, we're gonna go over here, where are you gonna be later?" I mean, this always happens. "We're goin' over here, where are *you* going?" You know, this sort of shit.

All the people that booze in this city, they can't go home. They got nothing to go home to. The skid row down here is loaded with people from all over Canada.

Everyone that came out of the residential schools basically looks at himself as a fuck-up. He doesn't realize that he *fucked up*. That "-ed" has gone out of the whole phrase and he becomes a "fuck-up." At first he used to blame himself for fucking up. But after a while he keeps dwelling on it and he starts looking around him and the way people look at him, then all of a sudden you're a fuck-up, you know?

But they're not alcoholics, that's the weirdest thing. They're not alcoholics. An alcoholic is a person that needs it every day. It's a sickness in which your body craves it. It's like smoking. You need nicotine to make your world go round. That is an alcoholic to me. Whereas the majority of natives that I know that drink a lot, they're escaping and they will turn to booze because of a situation in their life that has been altered drastically. It's their thoughts that makes their heart cry. It's not the booze. The booze just happens to be the pool they swim in. I've seen them without booze and I don't see them crawling around looking for the booze. But if you change the subject of their grief and rechannel that energy into more constructive things, where they have some worth, when you activate their mind into doing something constructive, they don't go looking for the bottle, so long as there's an alternative to the booze.

I can't see any of these people that have this booze problem make any great move of getting off of it. I can't. Not the ones that are committed to this city or urban centres. When they're sober, they look at their shame every time they cross a window and see their reflection in it. It makes them look at who they really are and they don't like that so they go find the nearest bottle. It's awful, but that's the way it is.

The problem is the honour. You gotta instill the honour and respectability of the native people. Their self-dignity has got to be reactivated again. They'll crawl off the booze once they got their honour back, their respect back.

When we're in our reserves, in our communities, we can beat it. 'Cause we have the strength of each other. But in the city you got to improve the lifestyles of these people. You gotta make them feel worth. You gotta make them *want* to be Indian. You gotta have their *heart* (*pounds his chest*) belong to them again as warriors — not as a bunch of scavenging idiots that this society created. We all know they used to be proud warriors. They are still *warriors*.

You ever seen them down on the drag there? Where they're yelling and squawking and screaming? You see how angry they are at cops? They know they're gonna get in shit, but they still do it. They're still brave. They're trying to be brave with what little they've got left and they're using booze to do it. And yet it's not the booze that's doing it. Society created the monster in these guys.

There's a few things that have to be made right first before the boozing will stop. We gotta answer the questions that made us turn to booze — the residential schools. Because what everybody's drinking on right now is the tears of humiliation. Not whiskey. Not beer. What they're drinking now is the tears of their own humiliation.

Figure it this way, over sixty thousand natives were processed through those schools since they started, and you got generation on generation just piled on top and now we're trying to figure out, "What is *love*?"

How in the hell are you supposed to know how to fuckin' love when you're not given love for ten months out of every year? It's obvious they don't know how to love. They ran away because they knew there was something missing. They didn't have it. Same thing with me.

You know something? I've had five wives. I have six children. My youngest is two years old. My oldest is twenty. I blamed all my wives for not following me in my quest for better jobs, better money. I used to get cheesed off and always say they wouldn't come with me.

I realized just a few months ago that was bullshit. I was running 'cause I didn't know how to fuckin' love. All these children but I don't know how to love. I was scared. Because I was never taught love. My parents died. Nobody loved me. Nobody ever held me. (*pause*) The only white man ever held me was a priest and the only reason he held me was he was tryin' to stick his cock up my ass. And they wonder why we drink.

The question is not, "Why do we drink?"

Ask first one other question, "Do you know how to love?" And you'll find a *very* thin line between them because they come from each other. You booze because you can't love and you booze under the guise of pretending that you can.

I remember trying to hold this girl when I was a young man and it was the most awkward thing. I didn't know how to. All I ever knew how to do was when I kissed somebody, I smacked my lips on their face and just hold on tight. I didn't know so much as how to kiss and I was seventeen! Yeah.

I used to play hockey for the Junior Greyhounds in Sault Ste. Marie. I could never get used to when I skate by, somebody tap me on the ass like, "Nice shot."

I used to go, "Get outta here. Fucking asshole."

Sure it might be through affection, but anybody laid a finger on me and I'd go, "Get outta here. Get away from me." My own teammates, I'd cross-check them and after a while nobody would dare touch me. Last time anybody put their hand around me, they wanted other than just, "Good shot."

Even when I went to college here, playing tennis, and the guy he's tapping me in the ass with his racket. "*Get away. Don't you dare touch me with that.* Who in the hell you think you are? A fag?"

You see native basketball players all over the Indian Centre and all over their own reserves. This generation never went to residential school. These ones are the lucky ones. Now you're seeing a little more comradeship, hugging and stuff. This physical contact.

Shit. We used to take showers like this. (*Stands and turns to face the wall.*) That's right. Because a supervisor is gawking at your cock and your arse all the time. That's what they used to do in those schools. Well, what kind of pride are you gonna come out of there with? I mean, really.

We gotta get our people home. We got too many detox centres and they're not doing it. They're not going to take these people off the street. Are you kidding? You know who they take? The people that got educations and fucked up. People that once had something and fucked up. But nobody helps these guys down here, under the viaduct, the ones on the street. Nobody helps them. They want out of the city, the majority of these people, but they got nowhere to go.

This is supposed to be our land and they find us there, in the most poverty-stricken places and situations. I mean, (*laughs*) give us a break. We're supposed to be the land-lords of this country, supposedly, and look where we are. Dammit, we're in deep shit as native people. We've lost our hearts. We forgot how to help each other.

If we gave native people some dignity, self-respect, they'll quit. So what you do is you put them back on the reserve, embrace them with open arms and say, "Come on, brother. We need you here. We need you to put our band back together."

Give them something to do. Tell them that their people *need* them. Make him feel he's wanted. "Hey, we *need* you. We need you to help us."

Nobody's ever called these people home. When they're down here, everybody just forgets about them. I'd like to call my people home, but you have to have a reason for having them at home. Once they're home you gotta have some place for them to *live*, some place where they can put their creative genius to work. And just give them something to do. But so long as none of their own people cries for them to come home, none of them will go home.

A couple days ago I quit drinking. I'm a boozer. I'm a guy that hides in it when I'm angry when things don't go my way. So once in a while I crawl into a bottle. I can understand the booze and then again I can't, so now I will stay to smoking pot.

I don't do any chemicals. I don't snort coke. I never have had a buzz out of coke. People give it to me and I snorted it, I shoved it in my arms, I put it in joints and smoked it. I never got a buzz. I'm trying to figure what it's all about.

And yet you give me a joint, tell me it's from Hawaii, *whoo-wow-jeez*. I'm already psyched out right into this already, man. (*laughs*) I'm already up there. That's the only thing I do now.

I don't believe in AA because I do not believe I should sit among other people and tell them my fuckin' story. I don't believe that. I think each person has to retain their own little personal *values*, their own sound reasonings that only belong to them.

A lot of native people that quit drinking, we haven't got a program by which we can participate, shy of sitting around becoming an *AA thing* like, you know, Alcoholics Anonymous. Who gives a fuck? You're still a person that used to drink. Why can't we just say that to each other? And this idea of admitting that once you're an alcoholic, you're always an alcoholic — that's a crock of *shit*.

There's enough heart and enough guts in the native. What makes us distinct from the rest of white society is *we have this heart, that's been with us for thousands of years. And we have it* (pounds his chest) *by which we can stop. Anytime.*

It can't be done with these little programs. It's nice to have these AA dances as far as socializing and stuff. It takes you out of the bars. But in reality it takes you face to face with other people that had the same fuck-up that you did. That's all it does. And every time you look at these other people, you realize you see yourself. Not as an independent entity, but as an entity of alcoholics. You're all back in the same big bag. I want to socialize, but where do you socialize after you quit drinking? I'm about to find this out.

I still got six beers at home that I can tie into any time I want to. And I look at 'em. It's gonna be interesting 'cause I've never had a problem by which I should quit. I've never quit *for* somebody. I'm quitting for survival, 'cause I know if I don't quit, my people won't survive, I won't survive. What I mean is my wife and kids. See, my wife, she has a very serious problem. She's not gonna quit. I have to forget about her and concentrate on my children. She won't quit.

If I let booze beat me, it's like a white man created another thing that beat me. But we're not white people. We're not weak. This is a disease that came upon us in the last two, three hundred years. It's new to us, but we should be able to conquer it. But it's not gonna be done through therapy and all this bullshit.

I just quit two days ago — until the next thing, and then what am I gonna do? *Go punch out somebody and I'll be in jail for assault*? Or just ignore it and let it really build up until I blow somebody away? If we bottle it all up, we become like time bombs until the fucking pile of shit you're carrying around behind you is so big it's starting to weigh you down. Then you're in trouble.

Natives, I figure, drink to hide truths, not fabricate lies. I realized that a long time ago listening to other people and what their excuses are. Drinking, to natives, hides truths of how they feel. That's what gets them into the deepest shit possible, there's too many truths. The truths aren't beneficial.

Like me. What am I going to tell my daughter when she's gonna say, "Jer, what's this about this Jesus and the God guy? Dad, what's this all about?"

What am I gonna tell her? "Don't believe that? It's a crock of lies?"

Or am I gonna break her heart and tell her, "Oh, you wanna hear Dad's side of what happened to him when he first ran into all this religious stuff? When he first heard about God and Jesus? And about the people that taught him all about them? And how they held their dick in front of him?"

What am I supposed to tell her? I'm not the only one stuck with this revelation. There's lots of us that's gonna have to tell these stories. *Do you lie* to protect your children? Do you? Or do you tell them the truth and *shock them all to ratshit?*

If you tell the truth and shock them, you're going to manifest a hate for this society, for white men, that'll go beyond what we consider hate now. It's not fair to them. It's not fair that I should have to answer these. I'll have to deal with how I'm going to answer. That in itself just might bring me back on the bottle, the stress of it. Am I gonna save the innocence of my child and *lie?* So consequently, lie to myself and crawl into a bottle because I'm lying to myself again? That's how I crawled into a bottle before, because I was telling *lies.*

It comes down to one thing. I'm gonna have to create animosity 'cause I'm not lying to my children. And then they're going back to school and tell the teacher, "My dad don't want me to know all about this Jesus Christ guy because he said you guys are full of shit."

And they wonder why we drink.

14

SOBRIETY

"What's most important to me is that I continue to carry on, one day at a time, to be sober and to heal and recover and live life to the maximum and be happy. I sure the hell didn't sober up to be miserable. I got a lot of healin' to do. But I'm gonna do it."

Hard-core drinkers don't usually quit drinking to become sober so much as they quit to escape the horrors of their alcoholism. In the same way that they drank to escape reality, they quit drinking to escape their escaping. Few people quit simply because they want to become sober. They quit because it is too painful to go on drinking. And after years of anesthetizing themselves with alcohol, they are forced to make a shocking discovery — that sobriety is more agonizingly painful, at first, than drinking ever was.

The first stage of sobriety involves the pain of physical withdrawal from alcohol. The physical pain is also accompanied by the emotional anguish of having to confront the problems that drinking created and the twisted causes that led them to drink in the first place. What makes it all worse is that it all has to be done without the painkilling effects of booze.

People who quit drinking, like people who undergo a major medical operation, have to go through a long period of recuperation in which the mind and body adjust to a new condition. The healing process can last the rest of the person's life. People who spent their entire adolescence and adult life as a blow-the-doors-down raging alcoholic, have to learn how to live sober and have to learn how to deal with the realities they always sought to escape. It's not easy for anyone to develop a whole new set of attitudes and behaviours, and it's that much harder for people who have been surrounded by alcoholism all their life.

Many people, thankfully, go beyond the stage that requires them to make the adjustments necessary to live a sober life. For them, simply being sober isn't enough. Instead, they make it their mission in life to become a better and more loving human being. They are determined to enjoy life and make the most of what they have. They are joyous, invigorating and fun to be around. For them, life and sobriety are great, fabulous, marvellous. They are wonderful company and beautiful people and the world is a better place because of them.

DANIEL is a shy, quiet twenty-three-year-old Cree. He began binge drinking when he was fifteen and "graduated" from a native treatment centre three months ago. He was interviewed in a motel room on his reserve in northern Quebec.

I never wanna even think of drinking again. I don't even wanna touch the stuff again. The thing that helps me not to, every time I think about drinking, I think about my culture — what kind of people I came from. I try to be in communion with the Creator also. Ask Him strength not to touch beer again. And I try to think as an Indian did a long time ago when there was no drinking. I try to be like that and to be proud of what I am. Proud of my nation as an Indian. And I try to be a spiritual person. I try to be as creative as I can be and as positive as I can be, even through hard times and bad times. I try not to walk on the path that I walked before. I'm living my life in a new direction now. A direction that has been chosen for me. A direction I was meant to go and not to walk the path of doom. I try to think of my role as a human being. I try to walk the path that God has chosen for me here on Earth. And I plan to stay on it.

ELSTON is the eighteen-year-old Stoney described in Chapter 9, who sobered up in a sweat lodge. He began drinking heavily when he was twelve years old. He was interviewed in a native treatment centre in southern Alberta.

I'm gonna try to stay sober, yeah. Probably will. It's pretty hard. All my friends are out there and they're still drinking. And if I graduate from here on the seventeenth and if I go home, they'll be bugging me with booze. That cycle will happen.

We had a weekend pass last month. I went home and my brother was there drinking. And he told me, "Come on, let's drink. I got nobody to drink with."

I told him, "No. I'm trying to cut myself down."

He got up, put his beer down. "Come on. Let's drink. You used to drink with us. You used to have weed and whiskey and stuff like that."

And I told him, "Yeah, that's the old me. Now I'm trying to live a new life."

And he got kind of mad and took his jacket off, took his cap off and he came up to me and he told me, "Come on. Let's drink. I got nobody to drink with."

He kept pushing me around and I pushed him back. I got mad and I told him, "Yeah, you got nobody to drink with, uh? I got no friends to stay sober with."

And he told me, "Just because you're at Stoney Medicine Lodge, you think you're tough and smart, don't you?"

I was gonna say, "I don't think I'm tough and smart," but he took a whack at me in my face. I got up and did the same thing to him. My sister stopped us. I told him to take me to the Lodge. So I spent the weekend pass here 'cause I couldn't face my brother drinking like that.

My friends are still drinking out there. I think they're gonna be the same way. I need new friends.

HAL is a sixty-five-year-old Tsimshian. He is self-assured and confident, with silver hair topping his rich brown face. He has been sober for seven years.

I won't allow myself to say, "I'll never drink again." I hope I won't. I'll sure do my best to stay sober by going to AA, by working my program. But I could not say I'll never drink again because we don't know. I've had a few temptations, you know, but I've put them out of my mind because I know the mental garbage pile that I come from and I don't want to go back to it.

I don't want to drink today. That's kind of a risky statement too, because who knows what the day will bring?

We got thirteen hours before the day ends and anything can happen. But for right now, I don't intend to drink. For the next hour I don't intend to drink.

SAM is a sad-looking thirty-nine-year-old Tlingit with long hair and a droopy moustache. He is a counsellor in Anchorage, Alaska.

I've been sober over seven years now and I've had a hard time. I have had times when I just want to say, "Fuck it," you know, go have a drink. Sometimes I get into these low periods where I wish I could be like I was when I was drinking, the feeling of not caring, that things didn't matter. It was easier. You didn't have to think a lot. Things weren't so complex. Sometimes I wish I was like I was, 'cause now I feel like I've become more aware of things and that gets difficult sometimes.

Through a number of workshops and jobs that I've had, I find myself in positions where I'm hearing a lot of hurts of other people, circumstances in their lives that are just truly unbearable. Hearing about family members dying, feeling the hurts, and feeling that I can't deal with this stuff, you know. Things just seem to get too complex and too hard to deal with and too confusing, where I just want to shut my brain off and just want to stop thinking about these things. Stop feeling these things.

And that's what alcohol and other drugs do. They shut my brain down. I miss that sometimes. Just being able to say, "Screw it all."

ALLAN is a twenty-five-year-old Peigan. He started drinking heavily when he was nine years old and he started taking drugs when he was twelve. He is now an addictions counsellor on the Blood reserve in southern Alberta.

People think when they're sober that it's gone. But as you sober up, there tends to be more problems and as those problems come along you gotta learn to deal with them. When you stop drinking, it seems like you got to start all over again from base one. Just like school, starting from kindergarten, starting a new lifestyle for yourself.

I've been sober for three years now, but I still got quite a lot of the past to deal with in order for the future to smoothen out. Every day I've been learning to deal with a lot of problems — marriage, financial, my job and just being patient with myself.

With the help of a lot of individuals and a lot of training that I received through my job, it's helped to smoothen the path out. It's showed me a lot of angles I never looked at before, a lot of the symptoms that I never looked at before. I thought sobering up was just that. But it's not. You gotta learn to get in touch with yourself.

TAMMY is a thirty-two-year-old Tlingit. She was sexually abused as a young girl and has been sober for ten years. She is now a secretary in Alaska. Tammy is thin, soft-spoken and a chain smoker. She drove her van to a picturesque roadside park for the interview.

I'm a super meticulous kind of person. I'm one of these people that there's a place for everything. I have the cleanest desk of anybody in my department and people are always making comments about that. I'm very organized and I guess that's a part of the disease, of feeling as though you need to be in control of all aspects of your life.

At times that's so good and I can feel that I'm in control of a lot of things. But then at times it's very confining, especially in terms of relationships, intimate relationships. That's an area that's really difficult.

It's kind of strange, because my professional life is completely different from my personal life. At work I'm very straight-up. When I start a project, I work on it until it's completed. I take things head on. I'm the kind of a person that if I have a problem with you, I'm gonna confront you right away. I'm not going to let it fester or make up stories in my mind. I need to be real clear where I am with all the people involved in my life at all times so I don't want to allow things to go by me without dealing with them.

For instance, I feel very offended when a group of folks are standing around and a woman walks by and a man wolf-whistles. I think that's inappropriate and years ago I never would have said anything. The same thing happens in women's groups, they make sexual remarks. I tell them, "Would you do that to a person's face? Would you go up to that person and make that kind of a remark to them? If you can't deal with it face to face, then maybe you should not be doing it. It's very rude and disrespectful."

At *home*, it's a different situation altogether. I have a really hard time communicating my feelings. I even get anxiety attacks to the point of losing my voice, 'cause the things that I need to talk about are at such a high level of anxiety for me. I have a really difficult time expressing myself in that way.

In a lot of ways I feel that I've made a lot of progress but I'm still an isolator. I don't have very many friends. I have very few female friends. And I completely stay away from men as much as possible. So I still have a lot of things that I have to work on. I'm aware that it can take me years and years still yet. I'm actually pretty amazed that I'm involved in a relationship. Not because I don't deserve it, but because I'm a very difficult person to be around. (*laughs*) I'm kind of like hot and cold running water.

SANNGIJUQ is a tiny, delicately featured twenty-nine-year-old inuk. She has been sober for nine months.

My life is totally, totally, completely and absolutely different. I wake up, bright and early, go to work, don't say things that I used to say, don't gossip anymore. I try to do meditation, go to sleep at a reasonable hour.

I guess an alcoholic person would find my life boring. At first I found it boring, but I have a lot of strength so I know what to do. I pray. I eat normally, that's like three meals a day. I take vitamins now. I look at myself in the mirror and appreciate what I see. I have a new outlook on life, oh yes, for sure.

Before, my life was looking for Mr. Right. I would find one and a few weeks or a few months later I would dump him. But now I find that I don't have to look for Mr. Right anymore. All I have to do is take care of myself in a nice, sweet and sensible way and just know that life will be all right if you just trust and believe in a higher power.

CHRISTINE is a short, bubbly twenty-eight-year-old Nisga'a with caramel-coloured skin, long brown hair and sparkling

brown eyes. She has been sober for four years. She was inter-
viewed in a Vancouver hotel room.

I hated being native. I hated being a woman. I hated my weight, my height. I hated everything about me. I thought if only I was a tall, good-looking white man (*laughs*) you know, things would be so much easier for me.

I was a wallflower. I would not talk to anybody. I remember growing up hearing that I was just a stupid drunk little squaw and I believed it, so I'd keep to myself rather than say anything.

Our family events were all based on parties and drinking. Drinking didn't *affect* our lives, it *was* our lives. We drank when we were happy, because there was a wedding. We drank because we were sad, because there was a funeral. We drank because we were angry and fighting with our spouse. We drank because our kids weren't behaving. We drank because it was Victoria Day. Any reason, any feeling, any emotion, *any excuse that we could find*, we drank.

Sexual abuse, wife battering, child abuse, child neglect, we didn't look at all those things in our family. They were in plain view and everybody could see it, but the alcohol helped to hide the shame. It was as if we had a pink elephant sitting in the middle of our living room and rather than find a way to get rid of it, we went around it, we avoided it, we didn't look at it, we pretended it wasn't there. Now there are people in our family saying, "Look. There's a pink elephant sitting in the middle of our living room!"

And some family members are still saying, "No. Don't look at it. Just pretend it's not there. Maybe it'll go away."

Whereas the people that are trying to sober up are saying, "Look, there's this thing in the middle of our living room. Why don't we try to get it out?"

It seems like there's more and more people in our family willing to look at the awful things that happened in our family: residential school, child abuse, sexual abuse, all that stuff. I know that for me, personal recovery has brought these things out into the open. Now I'm closer to my family. My brothers and I actually sit and talk and have a decent conversation. My mom and I are so much closer than we were before.

Now I am very proud to be native and I am even *more proud* to be a native woman. I try to show that I'm proud to be a native woman. I don't *tell* people that I'm proud to be a native woman, I *act* the way that I think a proud native woman should act.

My life is really different now. It's great. I have a *great* outlook on life. I have friends that I really love and that really love me and there are just so many fantastic things that are happening in my life. I'm still a party animal. I still go out and dance. I still have a good time. I just do it without the alcohol. I'm more outgoing than I used to be. I know I laugh a lot more. I feel a lot better. I'm more confident. I accept who I am. I still tend to tell stupid jokes. I love to talk to people. And it's because of those things that people are drawn to me. I know I like to be around people who are like that. I know that being sober is okay. It's *great*.

JANICE is a pretty thirty-two-year-old Cree-Saulteaux who lives in Vancouver. She wears blue jeans, cowboy boots, a silk scarf and rolls her own cigarettes. She has been sober for five years.

My eyes see clearer. I see lots more. I can lift my eyes *up*.

I never used to be able to do that while I was drinking. Everything was *down*. I couldn't look people in the eye. It actually sometimes would even hurt to lift my eyes up and look out and around me, so I'd look down.

It was easier to live in the dark than to live in the light — the light of *life*. The light of the world. The light of spirit. I was afraid of that. I was afraid that if I quit drinking, I would end up finding out that I had no spirit. And that terrified me.

It's as though I were another person, someone completely different. My mum used to say to me when she was angry, "You're so superficial. If you scratch the surface, you'd just get more surface." I never understood what she meant until I quit drinking. I was so superficial. I was concerned about the clothes I wore, so concerned of my image and yet deep down inside, ashamed of *what* I was. 'Cause I knew. I couldn't bullshit myself. I knew I was a boozer.

And *selfish*, that's where the superficiality comes in. When you live surfacely, you're only concerned about yourself. It wasn't till alcohol was out of my life that I realized there is more to this world than just *me*. The world does not evolve around me, and yet I used to think it did when I was drinking. So now I feel like I have some sort of *depth*.

Life is a hell of an adventure. Like I feel I can make adventures happen for myself. I can be *active*. I can go do this, I can go do that. When I was drinkin' I'd just scuttle from home to work to the bar. *Now, wow!* It's just wild, there's so much out there to do.

When I was first getting sober I thought, "My life is over. Everything is going to be totally boring now. I'm just going to sit around and not drink." And it *was* boring. The first year was like that because I was so focused on *not* drinking that I was immobilized.

When I was a year sober, I went into the pub with some friends. I'm sittin' there and about an hour later I'd had three pops, two coffees. I've *said* what I'm gonna say, I've *seen* who I'm gonna see and I'm hearing the *same b.s.* over and over and over from these people sittin' there. I thought, "For cryin' out loud! Is this what I've been missin'?" I've been gone a year and a half and these same people are sittin' in the same bar. They're sittin' in the same chairs, doin' the same thing, drinkin' the same drink and I just thought to myself, "*BOR-ing.*"

Now I go for walks, long walks in the rain and I enjoy the weather more. I'm not depressed with the rain. There were times when it was too sunny out, so I'd go in the bar and drink because it was cool and dark in there. Now I enjoy getting out in the sunshine. I even enjoy things I just used to absolutely *hate* to do, like taking transit. Now I enjoy being around people and talking to them. I don't have that fear of people anymore.

When I was boozing I used to think it was an adventure hanging out with bikers and dope dealers. I dressed like a tart, used too much makeup, real wicked haircut, real wicked mouth. I used to think that was life on the edge. You know, five o'clock in the morning, jumping on some guy's Harley in *March*, in the mountains with shirtsleeves on, and going down the road to do a dope deal freezin' my ass off.

I used to think I was real cool doin' that kind of stuff. And now, being sober, *that's* a hell of an adventure. *That's* life on the edge. It's good to be sober. I can't imagine any other way of living.

❧

JOHANN'S STORY

Johann is a twenty-seven-year-old Chipewyan whose childhood alternated between a trapline in northern Alberta and the skid-row streets of Edmonton. She is tall, thin and strikingly attractive. A student, she has been sober for four years. She was interviewed in her small two-room apartment in Edmonton.

I took my first drink when I was thirteen. It was lemon gin. I didn't mix it. I just drank it. I took a half a glass and I was drunk. The thing that I remember feeling about that very first drink was that I didn't feel. I couldn't feel anything. I was numb. Nothin' mattered. I was numb of feeling and all of a sudden I didn't care about anything. And not only that, alcohol gave me the illusion that I was okay. And all of a sudden I wasn't ugly anymore.

I drank for nine years, from thirteen to twenty-two. I did a lot of things when I was drinking in order to get a drink — prostitution, promiscuity. I did whatever I had to do to get that drink. And at the time when I was doin' these sorts of things, I didn't consider them as a means to an end, getting that drink, I considered it a way of life.

I became a lady drunk for a while. By a lady drunk I mean I had this really exclusive wardrobe and fancy clothes and I would sit in these really high-falutin' lounges with these high-falutin' people and talk about my second year of psych at the University of Saskatchewan, when in actuality I was a dropout and wasn't employed and wasn't in school.

Eventually my lies caught up to me. I never knew what I had said to the next person so I was really afraid. I didn't know what I said at what place so I didn't know what line of bullshit would catch up to me. I was too embarrassed to go anywhere 'cause when I was in a blackout, I didn't remember what I did or who I did it with or what I said.

I thought it was the people I was hanging around with, it was the city I lived in. So of course I did what's called the geographical cure. I packed my bags and went back to Fort McMurray, because that's where my family was and I thought everything would be okay. But the only thing wrong with that was that I brought me with me.

In Fort McMurray I was no longer a lady drunk. I began to be a biker. I was this mean, hard mama. I disposed of my fancy falutin' wardrobe and got myself a black leather jacket and tight-fittin' jeans and hikin' boots and hung out with the boys and the Harley-Davidsons.

The thing I liked about being a biker was the attitude and the lifestyle. When I was a biker, being a hard-nosed, hard, cold mama, so to speak, I could get as drunk as I want, get as stoned as I want and fuck everybody I wanted and exist with the attitude of "Who cares anyway?" If you don't like it — fuck off. Pardon my language.

The things that I did when I was a lady drunk compared to the things that I did when I was a biker were no different. I slept with as many people. I got as drunk as I ever did. I used any drug that I wanted to. But the catch was the attitude. When I was a lady drunk, I was trying to portray this facade that I was proper, moral, had values and was going someplace, you know? (*laughs*) The difference was the attitude. If you didn't like it when I was a biker — too fuckin' bad. And I let you know. When you're a lady, you can't tell people that and continue in the facade of being a lady.

My drunkalogue isn't important. What's important is why I drank and the effects alcohol had on me and my lifestyle. (*sighs*) On my mother's side of the family, I'm second generation to the cycle and disease of alcoholism. On my father's side of the family, I'm about fifth generation to the cycle and disease of alcoholism.

My late stepfather's side of the family, pretty near everyone has either been incarcerated or killed because of alcoholism. Very, very devastating deaths. And what is so bad about that is that my grandmother gave birth to these eighteen kids in the bush as a hard-working, good-lovin' traditional Dene woman, who had to watch her children die, one by one, from alcoholism.

My stepfather froze to death on Lake Athabasca coming back from his trapline. He was drunk. So he died from his drinking. I'm an adult child of alcoholics. My late stepfather was a drunk and my mother drank and I certainly did not have a healthy home atmosphere as a child.

My parents separated when I was three or four years old because of their drinking and then my mother met my late stepdad. When he moved in with my mother, I was about six or seven. That's when the maximum of the trauma began. I was a little girl at this time and there were seven little girls when all of this was goin' on. We were raised here in the skid row area of Edmonton and in Fort Chip.

My whole childhood — I was traumatized — was a state of shock. And I say that because (sighs) my late stepfather was a really violent man and he used to abuse my mother. I remember today that I gave up hope when I was eight or nine years old because this was the first time that we stood up physically to our late stepfather and fought for our mother's life.

There was always a fear, an element of intense fear. The fear was like always having a gun pointed at your head that you know was loaded and you're just waiting for the trigger to be pulled. So (laughs) there weren't very many calm, collected, breeze-through-the-day kind of things where you're just gonna come home and wonder what Mommy's cooking for supper. When I was a little girl I would be in a state of shock and fear, wondering if

Mommy would *be* home. And if Mommy's home, is she gonna be sober or is she gonna be drunk? And if she's drunk, is she gonna protect us from John? And if she is gonna be protecting herself from him.

We all had little hiding places — under the bed, in the closet — we'd all scatter off to like little mice whenever we'd hear them come home. We all hid until we knew for sure that there wasn't going to be any violence and then we'd come out. Otherwise, we'd stay where we were. Or if we were in bed, I'd stay in a paralyzing position of fear, never knowing what was going to erupt.

But this one time we could hear them coming and we knew they were drunk and we knew there was gonna be violence. We hid and we could hear the fight beginnin'. I can remember the screamin'. I can remember the yellin'. And all of a sudden I can remember the thud and the push and the thrash of my mother being beat and her fightin' back. And all of a sudden I didn't hear her strugglin' anymore. But I did hear the thud, thud, thud of his boots to her. I could hear the sounds of her body bein' hit and I knew she wasn't strugglin'. And we all ran to her and she was on the floor knocked out. Drunk. And blood. And he was beatin' her with his boots. That was the first time we stood up and we fought for her physically. We fought for her life.

One of the kids went to phone for the police and John ran away and the police got there and the look on their faces was, "Aw, shit! Them again." There was a look in their face that made me feel really ashamed, a look of disgust and anger too. It was just gross. They were almost pissed off that they were called again to our address in response to these children callin' that their mother was bein' beat. My mother got up and she was just full of blood and kids were just scurryin' around like crazed little animals in a total state of shock and fear.

Because of their drinkin', we were not nurtured. My mum fed us but it wasn't anything you could count on. You couldn't count on three or even one square meal a day. So I remember many times in grade two and grade three goin' to school and goin' into the coat room and stealin' other kids' lunches. And I 'member never, ever wanting to be at school.

School was a terrifying experience. My whole life was a terrifying experience but being at school was especially hard because I saw all these kids and their mummies and daddies made them food for lunch. And they had clean clothes. It was bad enough having to live the experience in my own home, but to have to go to school and to see what a dejected weird little kid I was, was even worse. And on top of that, not wanting to be in school because I had already assumed the role of the caretaker.

By the age of five or six or seven I had already assumed the role of taking care of my younger sisters and my mother. So I was always worried about whether Mommy's home and if she isn't home, who's takin' care of the baby, and so on and so forth. So school was not an experience that was very good for me. In grade seven I was beginnin' to act out so much that I was put in a special class for kids with behavioural and emotional problems.

I was the second-oldest of the kids. (*laughs*) We kind of had this hierarchy thing. John would beat my mom. My mom would beat my oldest sister. My oldest sister would beat me. And I in turn would beat my younger sisters. So we all kind of went around beatin' each other. And how bad the beatin' was depended on how bad you got your beatin'. It all sounds really devastatin' and it was. I do have some good memories, but they don't involve my mother. The memories of my mother are very traumatizin' and very painful.

I remember being sexually abused when I was about two years old. I don't remember the face or who it was, but I do recall the experience of bein' on a man's lap and him fondlin' me. Knowing at that age that what he was doin' did not feel right and was wrong. I was molested furthermore between the ages of two and five. My late stepfather sexually abused me between the ages of eight till I was eleven years old. And being that there was seven girls in my family, I wasn't the only victim.

As a child I was treated, what better way to say it, I was treated like shit. I was abused. I was not nurtured. I was not cared for in a healthy, functional manner. I was abandoned. Several times. I was always being moved around. I was never stable.

So I internalized everything. I wasn't a human being anymore. I wasn't a little girl. I was a piece of shit. And I internalized it. I took it within me and absorbed all of that abuse. I wasn't a little girl, I was this awful little thing. I was a victim.

My mother was aware that my late stepfather sexually molested us. But nobody phoned the authorities. Nobody phoned social services. Nobody phoned the police. Nobody told any authority that I was being sexually molested. So I was not protected and I wasn't, as a child, in any position to do anything about what was happenin'. I was totally and completely helpless and powerless, and finally at eight or nine, hopeless. I just internalized it all and became a victim.

I never had a childhood. I was always thinking like an adult. I was always havin' to be concerned what I was gonna cook for my younger sisters. I was always concerned about cleanin' up the place and makin' sure everything would be okay so that Mommy wouldn't freak out or so my late stepdad wouldn't have anything to be angry about. I was a little girl but I was takin' on the responsibility of my mother.

So that was the compact of my childhood and that was what I didn't want to feel when I took that first drink. I didn't want to give a fuck about whether Mum was gettin' beat up, about whether John was gonna come and fondle me that night. About whether we were gonna eat.

And when I was thirteen years old and I took that first drink, I got drunk and I had sex with my boyfriend that night. And it was kind of like the ultimate initiation of bein' a woman. I'm thirteen years old and I'm a woman now because I got drunk and I got laid. I was goin' based on what I saw, so to me I was a full-fledged woman at thirteen.

What that did was kind of made me a schizophrenic adolescent, of tryin' to function as an adult, at thirteen years old. Totally bein' responsible for myself, because I long ago decided that since nobody was gonna take care of me, well, fine. Fuck 'em all. I'll take care of me. And no authority, no parent or no adult could tell me what to do. I did whatever the hell I wanted to do. I was a rebel. I was not your average adolescent little girl. I was drinkin' and partyin' and sleepin' around and doin' all these extreme behaviour things.

I left home, got a job and boarded with friends and was able to feed myself, clothe myself and put a roof over my head on my own at fourteen. I was waitressing and when I turned fifteen, there was this mining company in Uranium City, and I was able to get a job as a cook's helper. I had a pretty comfortable income of $1,200 a month at fifteen and I took care of myself. I was able to function as an adult, but my emotional self was just a little victimized girl. So I would act like an adult with these peers that were ten years older than me and at some point I would become this little girl. It was always an extreme, a schizophreny personality.

I carried this victim state of mind well into my adult life. At thirteen years old, when I got drunk and had sex, what I remember was, physically, it was very painful. I mean excruciatingly painful. And what I did in order to cope with this was I numbed myself from the waist down. They could do whatever they wanted to do. I just didn't feel. Actually, sexually I never enjoyed the experience. It was very painful for me. But what I enjoyed was somebody was holding me. So I went on gettin' drunk and I allowed myself to be abused, sexually. I went lookin' for it. And the bottom line for me was, somebody was gonna hold me and it didn't matter what I had to do in order for somebody to hold me. And that first drink cured all of that. All of a sudden I just did not feel and it just didn't matter. So that was how my drinking career began.

Somewhere along the line, the community that I lived in, people saw what I did to myself and what I allowed people to do to me. Men, especially. So I began to get these wonderful little names like "whore," "slut" and "tramp." And, yeah, I believed all of that stuff.

I carried on this role right into my adult life, being a victim. And later on I caught on to this rage that I had because being the victim was no fun after a while. I then became the enraged person and what I did was I began to use and abuse and manipulate men. I kind of began this common-law career. I had twelve common-law relationships and one marriage between the ages of thirteen and twenty-four.

I thrust myself into relationships if I found myself attracted to someone. I went to extremes to get who I wanted. I call that part "Black Widow." I abused my powers as a woman and became a very seductive, manipulative, sensuous woman. I used sex as my bait as a Black Widow. I'd see my victim, I'd bite him, chew him up and spit him out.

I had all these unresolved feelings about who I am and all this internalized crap about this awful little kid. When people got too close to me, all of these feelings would start coming up and I didn't know how to deal with them, so I removed them completely from my life and I did that in a very abusive manner. I was physically and verbally abusive. That was my pattern. I thrust myself into these relationships without thinking about it and in the middle of it, would come up for air and go, "Oh my God, what am I doin'?" And then remove that part of my life and then become the victim and be totally helpless and powerless over my circumstances.

Anything went for me when I drank. I was never a social drinker. I drank from the word go to get drunk.

I figured I was doin' pretty damn good, comparatively speaking to my mother. I never allowed myself to be involved with a man who would physically abuse me. I allowed myself to be abused sexually, I mean, what else was I worth?

I was sixteen years old when I met my husband. I thrust myself into that relationship and went to extremes to make sure he stayed in my life. Four months after we met, he proposed to me and I accepted his proposal. A month after our engagement, I found out I was pregnant.

My marriage was beautiful. (*laughs*) I compared my marriage to being a female Fonzi from "Happy Days" being married to Richie Cunningham 'cause that was what it was like. When I first met my husband and I met his family, I asked him, "So, uh, you know, your parents drink?"

And he goes, "Yeah, they'll drink occasionally."

I say, "C'mon. Do they get pissed every now and then?" (*laughs*)

He's like, "*What?*"

"Well, do they ever get really drunk? Pissed? You know?" (*laughs*)

"Well, no."

So that blew me away. I said, "Okay, so they don't get pissed. So," and literally this is what I said to him, "Does the old man kick the old lady's head in every now and then?"

And he goes, "*What?*" (*laughs*)

And I said, "Does your dad ever beat your mom?"

And his face (*laughs*) went white and his jaw dropped but he knew damn well that I was dead serious. And he goes, "No, Johann. I have never seen my father raise a hand to my mother."

Well, that was proof that I had the right man. My quest for normality.

My very first Christmas with my in-law family just blew me away. They didn't all get drunk and fight and beat each other. Christmastime was always a very devastating time in my childhood. Other kids had parents that bought them presents and made a meal and Christmas bein' a really family-orientated kind of thing. It was never like that in my family.

When his family got together, Christmas Eve, at midnight, everybody was allowed to open a gift. I was in awe. I was in awe because (*cries*) they weren't drinkin'. They weren't violent. They were all together as a family. And I just couldn't believe it.

I didn't know what to go by. I went by "The Brady Bunch." I went by those kinds of programs that you see on TV but I was actually in a family that were doing these things that "The Brady Bunch" did. "Happy Days" and all that stuff. So I was in awe. Not only did they open a gift, they all gave each other a hug and wished everybody "Merry Christmas." And the spirit of Christmas, for the first time in my life, at seventeen years old, was alive.

The next day everybody got up and everybody was excited and kids were hustlin' down to the Christmas tree and openin' presents and I was right there with them. And the women, my mother-in-law, got out the turkey and all the fixin's.

After Christmas dinner we all opened our gifts and everybody did the family thing and this Christmas spirit was there, I said to my husband, I said "David, have you guys *always* done this?"

He says, "What?"

I said, "You know. Christmas thing. You guys always cook a big meal? And always get up at midnight and everybody opens a present and everybody gives each other a hug and says, 'Merry Christmas' and stuff like that?"

And he goes, "Yeah. As far as I can remember, this is how it's always been."

I was in complete awe. That Christmas was my Christmas gift.

The thing about that whole marriage was that it was a pretend game. I pretended, but it was difficult for me to be a good mother and a good wife. I mean, what did I have to go on? But I tried my best. I was a good wife. I was a good cook. I was very good in the domestic role as a wife to this man. I really enjoyed doin' all of those things. And when I became pregnant, I quit smokin'. Didn't drink coffee. Didn't drink alcohol. Didn't use drugs and had a really healthy, bouncing ten-pound, thirteen-ounce baby boy.

My marriage was my saving grace because all of a sudden I was introduced to a reasonably functional, reasonably healthy family. But the thing that was the end of my marriage was all that stuff that I internalized. The pain of that marriage was knowing that I didn't belong. They were a healthy family unit. But I removed myself from that marriage. I was really homesick and I went back to Fort Chip to visit.

I was eighteen years old at the time. I didn't smoke, didn't use drugs, didn't drink alcohol, didn't swear. I was very domestic, a good little homemaker, wife and mother. Although my life had changed with my marriage, my family remained the same. The insanity of my mother being beaten, the alcohol, the drinking, the neglect, the abuse continued. I always felt guilty through my marriage 'cause I had all of this good stuff and my sisters, they still had the crap.

At that point, bein' the caretaker, it was always important to me to be in total and complete control of everyone and everything. So I had the gall that summer to try to teach my sisters how to eat properly because I had learned how to eat properly, you know, using utensils, manners and stuff like that. Well, they didn't have that and I remember goin' home that time sayin', "God, you guys eat like dogs." I'm sure the only thing in their mind was that they were fuckin' well eatin'. (*laughs*) They didn't care how they ate or what manners they had, but here I was comin' from this together kind of mode and I was there to fix everybody and I was goin' to show them how to eat properly and how to have manners.

But I began to drink and I began to party and have this one affair and I began to smoke cigarettes and I went back to my husband a different woman. I was swearin', lit a cigarette, couldn't wait to get my next drink. My husband didn't know what happened. I began to view my marriage as me bein' totally undeservin' of the love that this man had to offer me. I didn't know what love was, because I didn't have the basis to go on. Love that was given to me through affection — this, to me, was really sick. My husband enjoyed showin' affection, it was all in love, but I would react the way I would react when I was touched that certain way by my late stepdad.

So I went about my quest to prove that I was undeserving and unworthy of this marriage and I destroyed it. I became abusive to my husband. When drunk, I physically handled him, verbally abused him. I went about it by getting drunk and sleepin' around and havin' an affair with my brother-in-law.

So that point on, from nineteen to twenty-two, my life consisted of gettin' that next drink, by whatever means I could. I left my husband and my son with him. I rationalized everything by saying, "Aw, I'm too young anyway. I've got too much life to live. Too many places to go and people to see and things to do."

My husband brought to my attention, at nineteen, that he thought I had a drinkin' problem. Well, the thought that I had a drinkin' problem never occurred to me. To me, a person who had a drinkin' problem was my mother or my stepfather or my relatives. Or any other Indian I knew. So on his recommendation I went to the Alcoholism Commission office in Prince Albert. I sat across from this woman in the office and she asked me, very solemnly, she looked me in the eye, and she said, "Do you think you have a drinkin' problem?"

Never had anybody asked me that. Never had I thought that. What the hell did I have to compare it to anyway? My drunk mum. But when she asked me, I had to ask myself and the answer was, "Yes. I think I have a drinkin' problem."

And when I said that, I felt like the weight of the world had been removed from my shoulder.

She said, "Okay, go to a meetin'. Of Alcoholics Anonymous."

So I went and I sat in this room with fifty people drinkin' lots of coffee and smokin' their brains out with cigarettes. And they all began to share their stories about their drinkin' and what scared me the most about bein' there was that I could relate to everything they talked about. I knew exactly what they were talkin' about. I might not have done the same things, but the feelin's they felt, I could relate to. And when they asked me to talk, I said, "Hi. My name's Johann and I'm an alcoholic." And I just broke down into tears.

From then on I went into a rehab centre in Saskatoon for three weeks. And this was how sick I was. I got out of the rehab centre after accumulatin' all of this information on alcoholism and I said, "So *that's* what's wrong with my mother!" (*laughs*) I was supposed to be in this rehab centre for *me*, for my drinkin', and I came out with the resolution that I discovered what was wrong with my mother. So of course you know what I did. I came back to Alberta and tried to fix my family.

And thus began Johann's career as a counsellor and caretaker to her family, to try to save her family from the depths of their alcoholism, especially my mother. And after that, from nineteen to twenty-two, I went through rehab two more times. (*laughs*)

My last drunk in Fort Chipewyan was pretty extreme. I was pretty wild, pretty wild. I literally had the community remove me from my home town. I literally had to go and hide so that people from my community could not find me. Let me say this: I wasn't the only person that was glad I sobered up. A lot of people were. I'm sure of it.

My last drunk lasted nine months, and in nine months I was sober maybe a month. By then I was a full-fledged everyday drunk, doing whatever I could to get that next drink. I was twenty-two years old and back in Edmonton.

I hated this city, because it represented the pain of my childhood. I wasn't coping very well. I came to the resolution that I was gonna be a prostitute full-time and I was just deciding what turf was gonna be mine. Was I gonna be one of the uptown girls? Was I gonna work with the rest of the native girls down on the drag? Was I gonna be one of the high-falutin' high-class prostitutes? This was what I had finally succumbed to.

Saturday night I was decidin' where I was gonna work. June 27th. I wasn't entirely sure that I wanted to do this and I wasn't entirely sure that I was an alcoholic, so I went out one more time and got drunk. I woke up the next day sick — hungover — and sick and tired of being sick and tired. Finally, I sobered up. And I've been sober since then.

I've been sober four years. I chose to maintain my sobriety through the twelve-step program of Alcoholics Anonymous and have been successful doin' so one day at a time. I don't feel that I could have stayed sober if it hadn't been for Alcoholics Anonymous because Alcoholics Anonymous helped me to learn how to live sober. In four years of being sober I've buried four people, and never had I the desire to drink.

What I'm really excited about today is that I know I'm a recovered alcoholic, that I'm an adult child of alcoholics. I've had to look back and discover my mother through a different pair of eyes and realize that she has internalized her own stuff via residential school, bein' beat for speakin' Chipewyan, her mother tongue.

Today my journey is a healing journey in sobriety. Today my journey is a discovering journey, discovering who I really am as a Chipewyan woman, discovering who I really am as a human bein', discoverin' who I am as a mother, as a sister and as a daughter. My Creator has brought many beautiful, spiritual people into my life that are on the same journey of healin' and recovery. And I see that my cry and my journey is my people's — whether they're Chipewyan, Cree, Cherokee, Navajo.

My people are on a journey of healin' so that we will rightfully take our place in this society and I see how I play a part in that today as a recovered alcoholic. I see that I am responsible when any sister comes to me in pain, in the depths of her hell. I can stand back and say, "Listen, honey. The strength you have is beyond your knowledge. Look at what you've had to endure. And you've survived. That strength will carry you on to anything that you want to become, to have a fulfilled, happy life today."

I especially extend that to native women, because to me what native women have had to endure in the last hundred years, compared to our pioneer foremothers who've helped the Europeans settle on this land, who've had to trudge their way through Riel and the rebellion, the strength and courage that native women today have is beyond our forefathers and foremothers because of the abuse that our men give them. They have to survive the odds of likely bein' battered women, likely bein' affected by alcoholism in their own family, their own community.

When I look at native women and I look at my life and I see what I've had to endure, I know without a doubt that I'm not alone. I am one out of many that are on this trek and this road of recovery and healin' and the longer into my sobriety, I realize that there are many people on this road to recovery.

You recognize that, "Yes, I am doin' this for myself." But when the Creator brings other women and other people into my life and somehow I am able to help them, I realize that I am not doin' it alone. I'm frontierin' a crusade of a people that are now awakenin'. I am not only healin' from the wounds of war, I'm healin' from the greatest,

greatest wounds that I spiritually have had to endure. And that's the wounds that are inflicted by this disease of alcoholism. Because they destroyed me and my family and my people to the depths of hell.

I affected everybody in my life and my family when I drank. They were severely affected by my behaviour, my attitudes and my actions toward them and toward life in general. But I am just as much affectin' my family today in my recovery and my healin', my behaviour, my actions and my attitude. Therefore I affect people in my life in a much more positive and a much more lovin' and a much more compassionate and acceptin' way. I just feel really elated and really happy about where I'm at in my life. Because where I'm at today is excitin', in healin', in recovery, in life. I'm healin' and it's excitin'. It's really excitin'.

But first and foremost, what's most important to me is that I continue to carry on, one day at a time, to be sober and to heal and recover and live life to the maximum and be happy. I sure the hell didn't sober up to be miserable.

I know that the Creator and grandfathers today have given me the strength and the courage to see the beauty in all that I have, to heal. I have a lot to be proud of today. It sure the hell is a far cry from the frame of mind of bein' a drunken Indian woman slut.

Essentially what it comes down to is, today I treat people and I treat life as a reflection of how I feel about me. And if I wanna get the maximum out of life now, I better feel pretty good about myself. I got a lot of healin' to do. But I'm gonna do it. I'm doin' it today and I'm livin' it and people feel it around me. I know that.

EPILOGUE

I began *Crazywater* by advertising in native newspapers, radio stations and friendship centres. I put up posters and handed out pamphlets. All of the ads asked the question, "Do you have something to say about native people and alcohol?"

Although I reached thousands of native people with my message, I was not swamped with replies. Many people, including some of the most articulate and thoughtful people I know, declined to be interviewed. Clearly, there is still a lot of reluctance to talk about this subject in the native community.

Fortunately, some people "interviewed" themselves and sent me their stories on cassette but I had to go out and get all the rest. The interviews took place all over Great Turtle Island — in hotel rooms, in cars, on skid-row streets, in bare-wall apartments, on the telephone, in coffee shops, on riverbanks, in offices, in treatment centres, and once in a Las Vegas casino. Some of the interviews were only ten minutes long. One lasted five hours.

The people I met represented a cross-section of native society — teachers, nurses, broadcasters, students, secretaries, bureaucrats, homemakers, writers, police officers, ranchers, librarians, pensioners, administrators, counsellors, engineers, cooks and real estate agents.

Some of the people I met were clearly in physical pain from the early stages of alcohol withdrawal. They were shaking. They were dirty, cut and bruised. Their speech was slurred and halting. Many of the people I met were withdrawn, suspicious or angry and wouldn't say much.

But I also found many, many people who impressed me deeply because they were so open and brutally honest; so willing to share the little they had; so willing to offer help, support and love to a stranger. Almost always these were the people who had quit drinking and found peace within themselves.

I knew when I started this project that I would hear some sad stories but I didn't fully realize how gut-wrenching the process would be. Dozens of times I listened for hours as perfect strangers poured out some of the most intimate and horrible stories I've ever heard. Many of them shouted with anger and cried with remorse. A few were so wounded by painful memories that they broke down sobbing and couldn't continue.

The interviews were almost as stressful for me. When people started crying, I usually resisted the natural inclination to lend comfort and support. Instead of reacting like any "normal" person, I had to force myself to concentrate on the job at hand. I had to take notes. I had to watch my tape recorder. I had to watch the time. But most of all, I had to get them to keep talking. Nevertheless it was impossible for me to remain detached. I often had to clench my teeth and clench my eyeballs to keep from crying myself. At the end of many painful, tear-filled sessions, I was hugging them, men and women both, and they were hugging me.

During the past three years I've had the chance to meet people who have survived some of the most depressing and devastating incidents I've heard in my life. I was awed to discover that many of these people were not beaten by their ordeals. They were not just survivors — they were winners. After years of pain, grief and misery, they were brimming with love and sincerity and bubbling with energy and enthusiasm. They were some of the strongest, most impressive and positive people I've ever met. The experience of sitting with these people and listening to their stories humbled me and cheered me. They are truly beautiful people. They are my heroes.